THE FINAL CUT

The truth about circumcision

Jonathan Meddings

ISBN: 978-0-6453682-2-2 (hardback); 978-0-6453682-0-8 (paperback); 978-0-6453682-1-5 (ebook).

Cover design and illustrations by Anne Donald.

Published by Jonathan Meddings.

www.jonathanmeddings.com

For James and Emmett

Contents

1	Cutting to the chase: an introduction	6
2	Not just a little snip	12
3	Cutting to cure?	25
4	A bloody mess	46
5	A view to a cut	59
6	Copy cuts	66
7	On religious freedom, rights, and the law	76
8	A religious rite that's wrong	90
9	Not so clear cut	105
10	Toward the final cut	115
	Notes	119
	Bibliography	136
	Acknowledgments	158
	Index	159

1

Cutting to the chase: an introduction

A distraught mother broke down in court, tears streaming down her face, her hands handcuffed and shaking, as she was forced to sign a consent form allowing her child's genitals to be mutilated.[1] This was the tragic end to a legal battle between a mother who fought to keep her child's genitals whole and intact, and a father who wanted his child's genitals cut.[2] The case was remarkable, not merely because the judge ruled the child's genitals must be cut despite one parent being adamantly opposed to it, but because while many will have reflexively imagined a girl, the child in question was a four-year-old boy named Chase.

Chase did not need to be circumcised for any medical reason. He had clearly expressed that he did not want to be circumcised. Indeed, he was positively terrified by the prospect. None of this mattered to his father or the judge.

Prior to being forced to sign away the bodily integrity and autonomy of her son, Heather Hironimus had gone into hiding with Chase in a last-ditch effort to protect him. The pair had evaded authorities for months by staying in a domestic violence shelter, following Circuit Judge Jeffrey Dana Gillen's ruling in favor of the father. The judge admonished Hironimus not to tell Chase that "she is or was opposed to his being circumcised."[3] Following her arrest for failing to appear in court,[4] Hironimus mounted a short-lived Federal Court challenge to the ruling, but withdrew proceedings because they appeared hopeless, and because she feared going to jail and losing custody of her son. And so it was that a court in the United States of America, in 2015, ordered the genitals of a young boy to be mutilated, and they duly were.

If this case had been about a parent running away with their daughter to save her from having her genitals cut, the law of the land would have offered protection. But because this was about a boy, Chase and his mother were instead forced to become fugitives in a failed attempt to save him from the same form of abuse.

Many people are outraged by the comparison I have just made, because they either think male circumcision is not a form of genital mutilation, or they think it is nowhere near as severe as female genital mutilation. They are wrong on the first count and confused on the second. Survivors of female genital mutilation, such as Ayaan Hirsi Ali and Soraya Mire, as well as many ethicists and medical and legal scholars, have drawn comparisons between various types of male and female genital cutting.[5] Of the four broad types of female genital mutilation, the removal of the male foreskin is most comparable to the removal of the female foreskin (yes, women have one too), which is considered Type 1a female genital mutilation. If we are to talk sensibly about genital mutilation, we must first break the taboo that prevents us from talking about when it is done to males.

The World Health Organization estimates that globally 30% of men are circumcised, of which 70% are Muslim.[6] That is almost 1.2 billion men missing the most sensitive part of their penis.

The legal battle over Chase Hironimus' foreskin made international headlines because it highlighted a confronting truth: a double standard exists when it comes to male and female genital cutting throughout much of the developed world, where the practice of male circumcision has become medicalized and highly profitable (see Chapter 5). Nowhere in the developed world is this double standard more consequential for young boys than in the US, where every year more than a million baby boys are strapped to plastic boards to have their foreskins ripped, clamped, crushed, and cut off. Some die or are left permanently disfigured because of surgical complications (see Chapter 4). Some experience lifelong sexual and psychological issues (see Chapters 2 and 4). All lose the most sensitive part of their penis and are scarred for life. Remarkably, most people – including most circumcised men – are completely unaware of all of this, but thanks to the efforts of activists and advocates, more and more people are waking up to the harms of non-consensual, medically unnecessary male genital cutting.

Most people in the developed world now accept that non-consensual, medically unnecessary female genital cutting is mutilation. They accept this, not because it was immediately obvious to everyone, but because for decades there was a concerted effort to educate people about the harms of female genital mutilation, and a subsequent push from the international community to eradicate the various forms of the practice. The list of countries that have explicitly outlawed female genital mutilation continues to grow, although it is easy to forget that the practice was not prohibited in the US until 1996, where an amendment preventing girls from being taken overseas to be cut only passed into law in 2013.[7] Despite these legal developments, a large number of states in the US are yet to update their laws to be consistent with federal legislation.[8] As it turns out, the fact female genital mutilation laws discriminate by only protecting girls means they are unconstitutional (see Chapter 7). Meanwhile, not only does the law in the US fail to protect boys, strengthened protections for ritual male circumcision were also put in place in 2016.

On 16 December 2016, then-President Obama signed into law federal anti-persecution legislation that extended protections to ritual male circumcision and animal slaughter, as well as to atheists.[9] One step forward (for atheists), two steps back (for animals and baby boys). It was only a year earlier while giving a speech in Kenya that Obama called female genital mutilation a "bad tradition" that has "no place in the twenty-first century."[10] It is ironic, to say the least, that a speech condemning female genital cutting was given by the leader of a country where more than half of newborn boys still have their genitals cut every year. The US also happens to be leading a campaign to circumcise millions of African boys and men based on debunked and disputed evidence that it reduces HIV transmission (more on that and the other medical arguments for circumcision in Chapter 3).

To those who do not come from a cutting culture, the reason for this double standard is obvious: just as many Kenyans see no problem with female genital cutting because it has been normalized in their culture,[11] many Americans see no problem with male genital cutting because it has been normalized in theirs. It's this normalization of genital cutting that causes many to refer to it euphemistically as "circumcision" or "just a little snip". These are euphemisms that should be rejected. The non-consensual, medically unnecessary genital cutting of any child, regardless of their sex characteristics,[12] is genital mutilation.

The only time "circumcision" is not a euphemism for genital mutilation is when the procedure is performed with the informed consent of the individual being circumcised, or in the case of minors too young to consent, for reasons of medical necessity. Such cases will by their nature be rare. A population-based study in Denmark estimated that a mere 0.5% of intact males require a circumcision for medical reasons before age 18.[13]

There are some who shy away from using the term "genital mutilation", preferring instead the more neutral "genital cutting", or widely used "circumcision".[14] In doing so they avoid any stigma that may be associated with a loaded term like "mutilation". However, many children's advocates and survivors of "female genital mutilation" refer to it as such, as do international organizations working to eradicate the practice. The reason for this, as noted in an interagency statement on ending female genital mutilation, is that "the word 'mutilation' emphasizes the gravity of the act."[15] This is a catch-22, because referring to "genital mutilation" is more effective at conveying its harms, but at the same time this has the potential to make some survivors of genital mutilation feel stigmatized.

While it is not my intention to stigmatize any victim of unwanted and unnecessary genital cutting, I often use the term "genital mutilation". I do so because I believe the term conveys appropriate connotations of harm, and because we will never see an end to genital mutilation unless people fully appreciate its harms. Also, despite the popular use of "uncircumcised" I will instead use "intact" when referring to anyone who still has the genitals they were born with, because "uncircumcised" implies a perfectly normal body part is abnormal and in need of removal. We wouldn't, for example, refer to women who still have their breasts as "unmastectomised", nor would most in the developed world refer to women who still have their foreskin as "uncircumcised". Still, it is worth remembering that until relatively recently "female circumcision" was a widespread euphemism for female genital mutilation in the developed world, and that this euphemism is still often used in parts of the world where the practice remains common.

...

The late Anglo-American writer, journalist, and orator Christopher Hitchens also criticized the euphemistic use of "circumcision". In an article on the subject in *Slate* magazine, Hitchens decried the practice of male circumcision, and argued that freedom of religion is not a license for child abuse.[16] Freedom of religion does not, and cannot, justify the religious circumcision of children too young to consent, because the absence of consent means such a practice is a violation of the child's right to freedom of religion, and indeed a violation of numerous other human rights (see Chapter 7).

Hitchens' article was the first I'd read on the subject of circumcision, and while I found myself agreeing with his argument, as a student of medical science at the time it occurred to me that a case could potentially be made for male circumcision if there were tangible and significant medical benefits that outweighed the risks of the procedure; benefits that at the time I'd heard about in the media, but not yet researched. In the decade that followed I did my research, and the deeper I dove into the medical literature, the more alarmed I became.

I discovered that the claimed medical benefits of male circumcision are at best negligible and at worst non-existent, depending on the specific medical claim in question. They are also beside the point, because while the medical benefits of male circumcision are debatable, that it violates medical ethics when performed on children too young to consent and in the absence of medical necessity is not up for debate. What's more, all the claimed benefits of male circumcision can be obtained by less invasive, proven means, such as condom use and vaccination; means which most, if given the choice, would consider preferable to having part of their body amputated.

During my research I approached the subject of circumcision with an open mind. On the one hand, like other intact men, I stand to benefit if the claims about circumcision are true, because the option to circumcise remains open to me, and with it the potential benefits that circumcision might bring. Admittedly, like most men I am quite attached to my foreskin (as it is to me), so the benefits would have to be substantial for me to consider being circumcised. On the other hand, most men who have already been circumcised didn't choose to be and are defensive when confronted by the idea that their foreskins were cut off by someone else without sufficient justification for doing so. This is understandable, because to accept that they have been mutilated is to come to terms with the realization that their parents, doctors, or religious authorities have wronged them in a deeply personal and permanent way. This is a difficult thing to accept because these are the very people in whom the most trust is placed, and who are turned to in times of need.

It is no coincidence that most men who are pro-circumcision are circumcised themselves, and yet more and more circumcised men are coming to the realization that a perfectly normal, healthy, functioning part of their body was removed without their consent and for no good reason. These men can be found on internet forums and at meetup groups the world over, and they're not happy,[17] which is understandable given they all had the most sensitive part of their penis permanently removed without their consent.

In my decade of research on circumcision, and through countless discussions with people who are for and against it, I have come to realize that the decision to circumcise is always based on one or more of the following six arguments:

- **the argument from health benefits** – "There are health benefits to genital cutting that outweigh the risks" (see Chapters 3 and 4).
- **the argument from aesthetics** – "Cut genitals look better" (see Chapter 5).
- **the argument from conformity** – "I want my child's genitals to match mine or those of a relative", or "Everyone else has cut genitals and I want my child/myself to fit in" (see Chapter 6).
- **the argument from parental rights** – "It's my child and I will do what I want to it" (see Chapter 7).
- **the argument from religious freedom** – "Stopping me from cutting my child's genitals violates my religious freedom" (see Chapter 8).
- **the argument from moral relativism** – "Even though I don't agree with genital cutting, I think people should be allowed to do it if that's what's done in their culture" (see Chapter 9).[18]

Writing this book has been an effort to respond to each of these arguments, which all abjectly fail to justify non-consensual, medically unnecessary genital cutting.

2

Not just a little snip

Many people think male circumcision is "just a little snip". Some even believe infants sleep through the procedure. Of course if that were true, they wouldn't need to be strapped down to plastic boards during it. Anyone who has heard the screams and witnessed the contortions of babies as they struggle against their restraints knows it simply isn't true that circumcision is "just a little snip" that some babies sleep through. The quiet ones are likely quiet because they're in a state of trauma-induced shock,[1] which isn't surprising when you consider that in addition to cutting, common surgical procedures for circumcision involve tearing, clamping, and crushing. Circumcision also involves the removal of 30–50% of the penile skin,[2] which if left to grow would average about 5 to 8 square inches in an adult.[3] This cannot be fairly described as "little".

How is it that so many people in the developed world came to view the genital cutting of baby boys as normal and harmless, but the genital cutting of girls as wicked and harmful? I believe the reason for this is that male genital cutting has been normalized in some places, as female genital cutting has been in others. How this normalization occurs is worthy of further consideration. Certainly, once most people have their genitals cut, views about cut genitals being more aesthetically pleasing take root, because that is all most people are exposed to. There is also comfort in conforming so one is not seen as different to the majority. However, to get to the point where most people have their genitals cut, people need to perceive the harms of genital cutting as sufficiently small to mitigate concerns over doing it in the first place.

Words matter

Words are powerful things, and the words people use to refer to genital cutting don't just signal their support of or opposition to it, they frame genital cutting in a way that influences how others perceive its relative harms and degree of normality.[4] Many associate "circumcision" with fewer negative connotations than "mutilation", which is why the former serves as a euphemism for the latter, but what exactly is the difference?

The Oxford English Dictionary defines "mutilate" as being 1) "to inflict a violent and disfiguring injury", or 2) "to inflict serious damage." The latter, more ambiguous, definition is usually only applied to inanimate objects such as defaced works of art. As for the former definition, the inclusion of the word "violent" is important because the Oxford English Dictionary defines it as "using or involving physical force *intended* to hurt, damage or kill someone or something" (emphasis mine), and most people who mutilate children's genitals have no intention of causing harm. Indeed, many believe they're doing the best thing for the child. There is no way then, according to this line of thinking, that the actions of such people could be labeled violent, because it is not their intention to cause harm. Of course, harm is nonetheless caused, from an act which can be construed as violent by victims of genital cutting, regardless of the intentions of those who had it done to them. That said, in the absence of medical necessity, my own view is that there is something intrinsically violent about the act of taking a sharp instrument to the body of another person and cutting away at it.

While it remains necessary to distinguish between an action and the intent of those who perform it, I think the act itself, and more importantly its consequences, are what matter most. I believe most people would agree, which is why most have no qualms referring to female genital *mutilation* despite the intentions of the mutilators most often being non-violent. Importantly, this means the fact most have good intentions when cutting the genitals of boys is not a valid reason for refusing to refer to this practice as male genital mutilation.

You don't have to agree with my definition, but throughout this book when I refer to "mutilation" I take it to mean "a physically harmful, and often also psychologically harmful and/or disfiguring injury", where to "disfigure" is as the Oxford English Dictionary defines it, to "spoil the appearance of" something. In my experience, people who disagree with a form of genital cutting being considered mutilation either disagree it is harmful or disfiguring, or both. While the matter of appearance is subjective, the matter of physical harm is not. Cutting healthy tissue always causes physical harm, regardless of any potential medical benefits that harm might be weighed against. This perceived difference in the degree of harm and disfigurement explains how the same individual can regard the excision of the female foreskin (or clitoral hood) as female genital mutilation, and yet regard the excision of the male foreskin merely as male circumcision.

On relative harms

Unlike male circumcision, the harms of female genital mutilation are widely recognized and condemned, even if not widely understood. As the ethicist Brian Earp has observed, when people discuss female genital mutilation they often think of the *most severe* forms of the practice, performed in the *least sterile* environments, with the *most drastic* consequences assumed to follow, despite this representing the minority of female genital mutilation practices.[5] By contrast, when discussing male circumcision, people often think of the *least severe* forms of the practice, performed in the *most sterile* environments, with the *least drastic* consequences assumed to follow.[6]

This perception that female genital cutting is always more harmful than male genital cutting does not reflect reality. The fact is that the harm caused by genital cutting, whatever the sex characteristics of the person being cut, exists on a spectrum. We already accept such degrees of harm exist for female genital mutilation, which is why the World Health Organization (WHO) classifies it into four different types,[7] in order of generally increasing severity from Type I to III, with Type IV inclusive of a range of other practices that themselves range in severity:

- **Type I (clitoridectomy)** involves the partial or total removal of the clitoris and/or the female foreskin;[8]
- **Type II (excision)** involves the partial or total removal of the clitoris and the labia minora, either with or without the excision of the labia majora;[9]
- **Type III (infibulation)** involves the narrowing of the vaginal opening by cutting and repositioning the labia minora and/or labia majora, with or without the removal of the clitoris;[10] and
- **Type IV (miscellaneous)** consists of all other non-medical procedures that result in harm to female genitalia, and includes "pricking, piercing, incising, scraping or cauterization."

The old classification of Type IV mutilations also included "stretching" and the "introduction of corrosive substances or herbs into the vagina to cause bleeding for the purpose of tightening or narrowing it", but these were removed in 2007.[11] Interestingly, reports released by the World Health Organization in 2010 and 2016 include stretching[12] and pulling[13] as examples of Type IV mutilation, indicating some inconsistency, and perhaps a partial reversal of previous changes.

As a look at what is considered Type IV female genital mutilation reveals, there are forms of female genital mutilation which clearly result in less physical damage than male circumcision. Indeed, prominent human rights advocates Soraya Mire and Ayaan Hirsi Ali, both of whom are survivors of female genital mutilation, have publicly acknowledged male circumcision as a form of mutilation that parallels some forms of female genital mutilation.[14] In particular, Hirsi Ali has said that male circumcision is worse than the "pricking" of the clitoris.[15]

It would be misleading to suggest that the relative degree of physical harm caused by different types of genital cutting isn't a source of disagreement. Equally misleading, however, would be to suggest that this point of disagreement matters. It doesn't, because regardless of the degree of physical harm caused, in the absence of medical necessity or an individual's informed consent, it is always ethically wrong to cut or otherwise alter someone else's genitals or sex characteristics, not to mention a breach of their human rights. More to the point: some being harmed more severely is not an argument for harming others less severely.

No doubt the argument over the relative harms of different types of genital cutting will continue, but it remains irrelevant to the wider argument of whether any form of non-consensual, medically unnecessary genital cutting is ever acceptable, and after more than a decade of studying the subject, I am yet to encounter a single scenario in which it would be. Perhaps that's because I believe that regardless of its degree, any *avoidable* harm to a child is unacceptable.[16] Those who disagree are left with the task of determining exactly how much harm it is acceptable to inflict. If one thinks the excision of the male foreskin is fine, then why not the excision of the female foreskin, or the pricking of the clitoris? This was the very question contemplated by the American Academy of Pediatrics (AAP) in 2010, when it released a policy statement on the ritual cutting of female minors, which argued that "it might be more effective if federal and state laws enabled pediatricians to reach out to families by offering a ritual nick [pricking of the clitoris] as a possible compromise to avoid greater harm."[17] The public backlash was as swift as it was unforgiving, and less than a month after its release the AAP had retracted its statement.

People protested the recommendation that the "ritual nick" form of female genital mutilation be permitted because they understood that although pricking is not as harmful as other types of female genital mutilation, that doesn't mean it isn't still harmful, nor does it mean it should be acceptable. This exact same logic can be applied to male circumcision. And yet despite it seeming self-evident to some people that all forms of genital cutting are to some degree harmful, many still see no harm at all in cutting their children's genitals. Indeed, due to social and religious influences, or perceived medical benefits, many parents truly believe they are serving the best interests of their children by doing so.

It is said the road to hell is paved with good intentions. Even the best intentions can have the worst possible outcomes. Most parents want the best for their children, but just because parents believe they are doing the right thing by their children does not, necessarily, mean they are. Actions can be harmful even if the intent is not for them to be so. The harms of male circumcision are indefensible in the absence of absolute medical necessity because circumcision is an irreversible, invasive surgical procedure that carries the risk of complications, causes scarring, results in loss of function of the excised tissue, reduces penile sensitivity, and may result in some types of sexual dysfunction.

Functions of the foreskin

The harms of male circumcision extend beyond the physical pain of the procedure and permanent scarring thereafter. Despite the widely held misconception, the male foreskin is not a redundant flap of excess skin, but rather specialized tissue with several important protective and sexual functions that are removed along with it by circumcision, including but not limited to the following:

- **Sensitivity.** The foreskin is the most sensitive part of the penis, with an abundance of specialized fine-touch receptors making it highly sensitive to sexual stimulation.[18] Intact men also find the gliding action during sexual stimulation very pleasurable, perhaps because of the complex sensory interaction between the head of the penis and the foreskin.[19] Circumcision removes the most sensitive part of the penis and reduces penile sensitivity.

- **Adequate skin coverage.** The foreskin provides adequate skin to cover the shaft of the penis during an erection,[20] which is why circumcision can result in painful, shorter, and curved erections.[21]

- **Facilitated intromission.** The foreskin facilitates intromission (the insertion of the penis into the vagina), with circumcision increasing the force required for penetration tenfold.[22]

- **Reduced friction.** Following penetration, the gliding action of the foreskin reduces friction, thereby reducing vaginal dryness. Studies have found that women are significantly more likely to experience vaginal dryness, and significantly less likely to orgasm with circumcised partners.[23]

- **Immune defense.** The inner foreskin is a mucous membrane that contains immune cells and specialized glands that produce a variety of antimicrobial compounds, which help defend against infection.[24]
- **Physical protection.** The outer foreskin protects the head of the penis and the inner foreskin, thereby decreasing chafing and preventing irritation and contamination.[25]

Of all the functions of the foreskin, its protective function is perhaps the most widely misunderstood. The fetal foreskin first appears at week eight of pregnancy and covers the head of the penis (or glans) by week sixteen, at which time the inner mucosal lining of the foreskin is physically joined to the mucosal lining of the glans penis.[26] In other words, the foreskin is fused to the head of the penis.

After birth, the cells connecting the fused mucosa of the glans and inner foreskin begin a slow process of "dissolving", eventually separating the foreskin from the head of the penis. The foreskin is not retractable until this separation occurs, so to circumcise a young boy the foreskin must first be ripped from the head of the penis.

When left to detach naturally, complete separation of the foreskin and head of the penis doesn't occur in most boys until early puberty, and sometimes not until early adulthood.[27] This is perfectly healthy and normal. Forcibly retracting the foreskin, on the other hand, results in pain and bleeding, and has the potential to lead to, among other things, scarring and infection.[28]

Unaware their young boys' foreskins are fused to the heads of their penises, many parents forcibly retract and wash behind their sons' foreskins; worse still, many wash with soap, further unaware that soap dries out the mucosa of the glans penis and inner foreskin, causing irritation and inflammation, and increasing the risk of infection. Soap causes the same problems for the vaginal mucosa in girls and women. Even as an adult, an intact man shouldn't wash under his foreskin with soap – clean water is sufficient. The use of soap doesn't present a problem for circumcised men, however, because without a foreskin the exposed head of the penis becomes chafed and dried out, causing it to harden (or keratinize),[29] and resemble skin rather than the mucous membrane that it is.

Some doctors, and other health professionals who should know better, are evidently also unaware of basic penile anatomy, with some advising parents to retract the foreskin,[30] and others forcibly retracting it themselves as part of their medical "examinations". A non-profit organization called

Doctors Opposing Circumcision deals with over 100 requests for first aid and assistance filing complaints for premature, forcible foreskin retraction each year.[31] Just how widespread premature, forcible foreskin retraction is remains unknown, but according to one estimate there are 100,000 cases each year in the US alone.[32] This number of course excludes the forcible retraction that occurs at the start of the more than one million circumcisions performed in the US each year.

Circumcision reduces penile sensitivity and may cause sexual dysfunction

The foreskin is the most sensitive part of the penis and has important sexual functions, so it may strike readers as obvious that cutting it off reduces penile sensitivity and causes sexual dysfunction. Remarkably, however, the evidence of circumcision's impact on penile sensitivity is mixed, and seemingly as many studies conclude it has no effect on sensitivity, or even that it *increases* sensitivity, as those that conclude that sensitivity is reduced. The evidence is also mixed as to whether circumcision causes different types of sexual dysfunction, such as impotence, diminished sexual pleasure or desire, difficulty reaching orgasm, or premature ejaculation. Having reviewed the medical evidence, I think circumcision clearly reduces penile sensitivity, and it is quite possible that it causes some types of sexual dysfunction. But before we walk through that medical minefield, it is necessary to understand some anatomy.

Free nerve endings in skin are involved in sensing heat, cold, deep pressure, or pain.[33] Touch receptors are involved in different sensations, and although there are many different types of touch receptors, the ones we are primarily concerned with are the corpuscular receptors (or corpuscles), which are involved in sensing fine touch (Meissner's corpuscles) or pressure and vibration (Pacinian corpuscles). Both the clitoris and the penis – including the head of the penis – contain erectile tissue. However, this erectile tissue is lacking in the head of the clitoris.[34] This anatomical difference might explain why the head of the clitoris has, on average, more corpuscles (4.52 per millimeter) than the head of the penis (1.29 per millimeter).[35] As a point of comparison, there is an average of 2.7 corpuscles per millimeter of skin on the human hand.[36] It is this difference in the density of corpuscles that explains why the head of the clitoris is more sensitive than the head of the penis. The lack of corpuscles in the head of the penis has been noted before, with free nerve endings exceeding them by a ratio of 10 : 1.[37] Indeed, the only part of the body with fewer fine-touch receptors than the head of the penis is the heel of the foot.[38] If this fact isn't enough to drive home that the head of the penis is simply insensitive to fine touch, then let me put it another way: the threshold for touch in the head of the penis is the pain threshold.[39] By comparison, the male foreskin, like the fingertips, has an abundance of Meissner's corpuscles that are highly sensitive to fine touch.[40]

Given that we know the foreskin is highly sensitive to fine touch and the head of the penis is not, you'd expect the results of investigations on circumcision status and penile sensitivity to show a clear negative impact. So why have their results been mixed? One major reason for this is that most studies have relied on subjective survey-based responses. This limitation can be found in studies that have reported erectile dysfunction, reduced penile sensitivity, and reduced masturbatory pleasure following circumcision,[41] as well as studies that have reported no such deleterious effects.[42] Many men have also proved incapable of correctly identifying their circumcision status,[43] so any study relying on men to correctly identify their circumcision status is likely to have compromised results from the start.

Very few studies on penile sensitivity to date have accounted for both the subjective nature of self-reporting, and the inability of men to correctly identify their circumcision status, despite both being obvious sources of error. One study that did not suffer from these sources of error quantitatively compared fine-touch pressure threshold differences between circumcised and intact adult men.[44] It found that the head of the penis in intact men was significantly more sensitive than in circumcised men, and that the circumcision scar was the most sensitive part of the circumcised penis, but that it was still significantly less sensitive than several regions of the intact penis that are removed by circumcision.[45]

There are four main methodological advantages that made the results of this study more reliable than others. First, it used an objective measure rather than a subjective one (i.e., it applied a known pressure and asked men about the sensation they felt, rather than asking them how they rated their sensitivity on a scale without a point of reference). Second, it recorded the sensation men reported feeling at the time, not what they thought they remembered feeling at some point in the past when answering a survey in the present. Third, because a physician measured the fine-touch sensitivity, it allowed for proper identification of the circumcision status of the subjects. And fourth, this study recorded fine touch measurements from 19 different sites on the penis, including several from different areas of the foreskin. Still, as the researchers of the study noted, sensation involved in fine touch is likely more dynamic than can be assessed by a static measurement of a pressure threshold at any given point.[46] This limitation is not reason to dismiss the study's results; rather it suggests that the richness of sensation enabled by the corpuscle-dense regions of the foreskin is likely even greater than was, or indeed can, be measured.

Of the few other quantitative sensory studies that have been performed, those that reported circumcision caused no reduction in penile sensitivity either did not bother to test the sensitivity of the foreskin (choosing instead to only test the sensitivity of the head of the penis),[47] or they only tested a single site on the outer foreskin tissue.[48] That these studies either ignored the most sensitive part of the penis, or only took a selective measurement of it, explains why they found no significant difference in penile sensitivity between circumcised and intact men. Curiously, one of these studies found the outer foreskin to be more sensitive than any of the other sites tested, yet counter-intuitively concluded that there are "minimal long-term implications to penile sensitivity exist as a result of the surgical excision of the foreskin."[49] As Brian Earp said in his critique of this study, drawing such a conclusion from its results is "akin to stating that the neonatal removal of the little finger is not associated with changes in hand sensitivity ... Given that the little finger is part of the hand [and] is sensitive in its own right, such [a statement] cannot logically be true."[50]

Other studies in need of critical analysis are two sexual function studies, one conducted in Uganda,[51] and the other in Kenya,[52] which the American Academy of Pediatrics referred to as being of "good quality", and which formed the cornerstone of its conclusion that "circumcision does not appear to adversely affect penile sexual function/sensitivity or sexual satisfaction."[53] It so happens these two studies were run in tandem with trials in Uganda and Kenya that aimed to determine if male circumcision reduces female-to-male HIV transmission. As we will see in the next chapter, both HIV trials are deeply flawed, and unfortunately the two sexual function studies are flawed as well. Speaking of their results, Robert Van Howe, a professor of medicine at Central Michigan University, said "their rates of sexual dysfunction were 6 to 30 times lower than reported in other countries [so] the men in these studies, if the results are to be believed, are having the best sexual experiences on the planet."[54] Or, rather more likely, the surveys used in these studies were insensitive and flawed.[55] Morten Frisch of the Department of Epidemiology Research at the Statens Serum Institut in Copenhagen, having obtained the questionnaires from the authors of the Ugandan and Kenyan sexual function studies, found that several questions were so vague they did not even provide a clear distinction between premature ejaculation and difficulty reaching orgasm, or sexual problems related to intercourse and masturbation.[56] In other words, the survey questions were so vague that they were unable to capture possible differences between circumcised and not-yet circumcised participants.[57] Flawed questions in what were both survey-based studies – not off to a great start.

Another problem with the Kenyan and Ugandan studies is that condoms were made freely available to participants (both circumcised and intact), but both studies failed to mention if the type of condom used was controlled for (presumably it wasn't), or if subjects also used their own condoms (presumably many did). Due to this oversight, we have no way of knowing if some subjects were provided with, or at any point used, "thin" condoms, which are specifically marketed to men because being thinner they allow for greater sensation. It is surprising that a variable with such an obvious potential to impact results was not identified, let alone any attempt made to control for it.

Although it doesn't relate to penile sensitivity or sexual function, it's also worth noting the authors of the Kenyan study reported that circumcised men found condoms increasingly "easier to use" from 6 to 24 months, appearing to farcically imply condom use was easier because of their circumcision.[58] If this was the intended implication, it is a rather bizarre one. As an intact man I've never had any trouble using a condom, and I think it is reasonable to assume that whether circumcised or not, most other adult men who have used a condom before don't suffer any great difficulty using them either. As for the likely reason men participating in the Kenyan study found condoms easier to use over time, 63% of circumcised and 63% of intact participants in the HIV trial that this sexual function trial was piggybacking on hadn't used a condom in the six months before the trial started.[59] I suspect many had never used a condom before, and if so, the fact they were repeatedly counseled about how to use condoms during the trial would explain why participants in the circumcised group found condoms progressively easier to use. One would expect the same result for intact men in the control group, but the researchers either chose not to collect, or not to publish the data on ease of condom use in the intact control group.

The debate in the medical literature over the effect of circumcision on penile sensitivity is ongoing. It nonetheless defies logic, common sense, and the best available evidence that circumcision, in its removal of highly sensitive foreskin tissue and subsequent hardening (or keratinization) of the head of the penis, should result in anything other than a reduction of penile sensitivity.

If circumcision does indeed reduce penile sensitivity, this might contribute to a decline in condom use. Despite this serious concern, some circumcision proponents have flippantly argued that circumcision reducing sensitivity is a good thing, because it helps men last longer in bed.[60] There are a few things to be said of this. First, that men will prefer sex to last longer if it comes at the expense of more pleasurable sex and masturbation is a massive assumption. Second, there are alternatives for men to last longer during sex other than mutilating their genitals: they could, for example, talk through their issues with a sex therapist, or speak with their general practitioner about the possibility they suffer from premature ejaculation and discuss their treatment options. Third, whether the desensitizing effects of circumcision will help men last longer in bed depends on whether they end up suffering impotence or premature ejaculation because of circumcision. This last point is contentious and requires an understanding of a bit more anatomy.

Previously thought to be purely psychological in origin, primary (or lifelong) premature ejaculation, which refers to a man's chronic inability to control his ejaculatory reflex from the beginning of his sexual life, is now thought to be genetic and neurobiological in origin. By comparison, secondary (or acquired) premature ejaculation affects men who have not previously suffered from it, and is psychological, or the result of some underlying disorder (such as an overactive thyroid gland or swollen and inflamed prostate).[61]

In patients with a suspected neurological cause of premature ejaculation, bulbocavernosus reflex testing is often useful. The test involves applying an electrical stimulus to a particular nerve of the penis and recording the response of the bulbocavernosus muscle[62] (hence the corresponding name of the reflex). While this muscle plays a small role in maintaining a rigid erection,[63] its role is too small to make bulbocavernosus reflex testing a useful diagnostic tool for erectile dysfunction.[64] More importantly, the rhythmic contraction of the bulbocavernosus muscle, along with other muscles, is necessary to facilitate ejaculation.[65] What is interesting to note is that circumcised men have a diminished bulbocavernosus reflex, with one study finding the reflex was "clinically non-excitable" for 73% of men in the circumcised group, compared to just 8% in the intact control group.[66]

The apparent dampening of the bulbocavernosus reflex in circumcised men may explain why some studies have shown circumcision improves intravaginal latency ejaculation time,[67] which is the technical term for how long a man can last before reaching orgasm during vaginal sex. In other words, circumcised men have more difficulty reaching orgasm than intact men.[68]

Harder to explain is how some studies indicate circumcision makes it more difficult to reach orgasm, while others have indicated circumcised men are more likely to experience premature ejaculation.[69] Specifically, how could circumcision simultaneously make it more difficult for some men, and too easy for others, to reach orgasm? To make any sense of these conflicting results an understanding of the suspected causes of premature ejaculation is needed.

Among the known causes of lifelong premature ejaculation is genetic predisposition.[70] If the cause is largely genetic in origin it is unlikely circumcision would influence premature ejaculation either way. Unfortunately, all the studies on circumcision and premature ejaculation conducted so far have not determined if their subjects were genetically predisposed to premature ejaculation, so it remains unclear if circumcision is a potential cause of premature ejaculation in cases without a genetic component. Hyperexcitability of the bulbo-cavernosus reflex is another suspected cause of lifelong premature ejaculation.[71] Hypersensitivity of the penis may,[72] or may not,[73] be another cause. On the assumption that penile hypersensitivity is a cause, some have proposed circumcision as a treatment for premature ejaculation for its ability to reduce penile sensitivity.[74] However, circumcision remains unproven as a treatment option for premature ejaculation and is therefore not recommended.[75] As there is no definitive answer on whether circumcision causes or alleviates premature ejaculation, or makes no difference, most men refuse circumcision as a treatment for premature ejaculation on the basis that it is an irreversible, costly body modification that can cause complications, and offers no guarantee of success.[76]

To complicate things further, premature ejaculation may sometimes result from a history of erectile dysfunction, with some men reporting that their rapid ejaculation is sometimes due to their concern they'll lose their erection before they orgasm.[77] And to complicate things even more, since sexual dysfunction often has a psychological cause, whether circumcision is perceived to enhance or diminish sexual function will depend to some extent on whether individuals think it will.

All things considered, it appears most likely that circumcision often makes ejaculation more difficult by diminishing the bulbocavernosus reflex, that it sometimes results in erectile dysfunction due to reduced penile sensitivity and psychological impacts, and that while circumcision itself probably doesn't directly cause premature ejaculation, some circumcised men might experience premature ejaculation secondary to their erectile dysfunction.

...

The foreskin is not a useless flap of skin – it is specialized tissue with important sexual and protective functions. The removal of the highly sensitive foreskin tissue results in the loss of its functions, reduces penile sensitivity, can reduce erectile length, and may even cause some types of sexual dysfunction. In addition to its physical harms, many men experience psychological harms following the trauma of circumcision (more on that in Chapter 4). Circumcision is not "just a little snip". It is an invasive, harmful, irreversible surgical procedure with serious lifelong consequences.

3

Cutting to cure?

No professional organization of medical doctors anywhere in the world recommends routine infant circumcision, yet every year millions of newborn boys lose their foreskins to the procedure. Qualified support for male circumcision is limited to the World Health Organization (WHO), the Joint United Nations Programme on HIV/AIDS (UNAIDS), and the United Nations International Children's Emergency Fund (UNICEF). These organizations do important work, but none of them are primarily organizations of medical doctors – they are bureaucratic bodies concerned with public health. The qualified support of the WHO, UNAIDS and UNICEF for male circumcision is strictly limited to HIV endemic regions of sub-Saharan Africa. Unfortunately, their support for the mass circumcision of millions of African boys and men to reduce HIV transmission rests largely on three randomized control trials conducted in Africa, which as we will soon see, suffered from flawed methods that served to grossly exaggerate their results.

Circumcision proponents often claim that the American Academy of Pediatrics (AAP) also recommends routine infant male circumcision. It does not. In 1999, the AAP released a policy statement that said there are potential medical benefits to male circumcision, but that they are not sufficient to recommend the procedure be performed routinely on infants.[1] Then in 2012, the AAP released an updated policy statement that said the benefits of circumcision outweigh the risks, but still fell short of recommending it as a routine procedure.[2] The US is the only country in the Anglosphere that still routinely circumcises the majority of newborn boys, and its relevant peak medical body doesn't even recommend the practice.

That said, the AAP has displayed a relatively favorable view of circumcision in stating the benefits outweigh the risks. This view is out of step with the international medical consensus that the benefits *do not* outweigh the risks. It is so out of step, in fact, that dozens of eminent doctors from around the world published a paper in *Pediatrics* (the official journal of the AAP) that was highly critical of the AAP's 2012 policy statement.

The paper charged the AAP with "cultural bias" and concluded that, in addition to offering no compelling health benefits, causing postoperative pain, and having the potential for serious long-term consequences, non-therapeutic circumcision breaches the rights of the child and conflicts with the Hippocratic oath (*Primum non nocere:* First, do no harm).[3]

Following on from the AAP's 2012 policy statement, in December 2014 the United States Centers for Disease Control (CDC) released draft guidelines – which have yet to be followed by any official policy position – titled, *Recommendations for providers counseling male patients and parents regarding male circumcision and the prevention of HIV, STIs, and other health outcomes* (hereafter the CDC guidelines). The CDC guidelines cited the AAP position that the benefits of circumcision outweigh the risks, but also stopped short of recommending routine infant circumcision. Instead, it was merely recommended that parents and patients should be counseled on the risks and benefits of male circumcision. This should be happening anyway but, as the need for this recommendation reveals, isn't occurring in many cases.

As with the AAP policy statement, there has been no shortage of criticism of the CDC guidelines.[4] Some of the main criticisms of the CDC guidelines can be summarized as follows:

1) They ignore the legal and bioethical consensus that unnecessary surgery – particularly that which removes healthy tissue without consent – constitutes a harmful act in and of itself, even if the surgery is executed flawlessly.

2) Despite emphasizing the need for parents and men to be informed about the benefits and risks of circumcision, no recommendations are made regarding the need to inform them of the physiology and functions of the foreskin, and without this information, it is impossible to truly provide informed consent.

3) The CDC guidelines state, as many supporters of infant circumcision have also argued, that "neonatal male circumcision is, safer, and heals more rapidly than circumcision performed on older boys, adolescent males, and men, and is less expensive."[5]

There are two problems with this third point (three if you count the rogue comma). First, it ignores the fact there's debate about whether infant circumcision really has fewer complications (and is therefore safer). Some have argued that complications in infants are underreported, because unlike older children and adults, infants lack the ability to complain.[6] Second, simply stating that infant circumcision is less costly glosses over the reason why: adult circumcision is more costly due to the use of general anesthesia, which is avoided in young children because it can cause life-threatening respiratory problems, especially in infants.[7] This means that when the surgery is performed on infants, at worst it is performed without pain control, and at best with sub-optimal pain control, meaning costs are driven down at the expense of humane treatment.[8]

Clearly there are many problems with the CDC guidelines, but by far the greatest problem for the CDC, or any organization that supports male circumcision for its supposed health benefits – which range from preventing penile cancer and urinary tract infections, to reducing transmission of sexually transmissible infections – is that these benefits are either unproven, greatly exaggerated, or obtainable using vaccines and condoms instead. These are methods that most would consider preferable to having part of their genitals cut off, particularly given that in addition to being more effective they also remain necessary even if you've been circumcised. That's why, despite calling for the mass circumcision of African boys and men in a desperate attempt to combat HIV, the WHO and UNAIDS concede it only provides a partial effect, and that it needs to be used in conjunction with far more effective and proven means of prevention, such as condom use.

The remainder of this chapter will explore the full range of medical arguments for circumcision, revealing how the procedure is rarely medically justified. Before we navigate the medical arguments, however, let us briefly look at the history of circumcision as a "medical" procedure.

A brief history of medical circumcision

Many articles that support male circumcision, including those in medical journals, begin by informing readers that it is the oldest surgical procedure known, and has been practiced by many ancient cultures. However, circumcision as a medical procedure is a relatively recent phenomenon.

Male circumcision was first introduced as a medical procedure in the eighteenth century as a desperate and ineffective last resort to treat severe venereal infection, which often resulted in scabs that fused the foreskin to the head of the penis.[9] Following this, things got a little out of hand, and doctors started claiming circumcision prevented or cured a long list of ailments, ranging from sexual diseases such as syphilis, to sexual disorders such as impotence and sterility, and curiously even neurological disorders such as epilepsy, which prepubertal orgasms were misinterpreted as being a sign of.[10]

The promotion of circumcision as a treatment or cure was by no means limited to real medical conditions. Indeed, it was widely promoted as a way of preventing masturbation, which was thought to result in numerous ills, and as a way of curing what were once *perceived* sexual disorders, such as homosexuality, as well as the medical understanding of "spermatorrhea" at the time, in which almost any loss of semen outside of heterosexual marital intercourse was considered pathological.[11]

It wasn't until the early nineteenth century that male circumcision took hold as a *routine* procedure in Britain and America, performed for so-called 'medical' reasons like preventing masturbation. It was thought boys would not masturbate if the most sensitive part of their penis had been removed. Ironically, not only did circumcision fail to prevent men from masturbating, by dulling sensation it succeeded only in making them work harder at it.

Adding not mere insult, but rather immense pain to injury, circumcisions were frequently performed without anesthetic, because it was believed "the brief pain attending the operation will have a salutary effect on the mind, especially if it be connected with the idea of punishment."[12]

Although less common, "female circumcision" – the surgical removal of the female foreskin and often also the clitoris – was also recommended as a preventative and curative measure for female masturbation.[13] There is debate among medical historians about how doctors viewed the clitoris at the time. On the one hand, there are those like Rachel Maines, who argued that many physicians misunderstood the role of the clitoris in arousal to orgasm "since its function contradicted the androcentric principle that only an erect penis could provide sexual satisfaction to a healthy, normal adult female."[14] On the other hand, there are those like Sarah Rodriguez, who take the view that physicians "respected the importance of clitoral stimulation for healthy sexuality while simultaneously recognizing its role as a cause and symptom in cases of insanity that were tied to masturbation."[15] Whatever the case, the physicians were clearly far off the mark.

Modern medicine has come a long way since doctors first started trying to cut their way to a cure, and yet male circumcision, unlike "female circumcision", remains a common procedure (and a common euphemism) in many parts of the developed world today; although it must be remembered that "female circumcision" remained accepted by the medical community in America until well into the 1960s. To provide but one particularly apt example of the medical profession's ignorance of the harms of female genital cutting at the time, in 1959, Californian physician W. G. Rathmann published a paper titled, *Female Circumcision:*

Indications and a New Technique. In it he detailed a new device for the excision of the female foreskin, and argued that among other things its removal is advisable when a woman is "quite adipose" (meaning fat), or when "the husband is unusually awkward or difficult to educate [such that one needs to make] the clitoris easier to find."[16] These reasons for cutting off the female foreskin, absurd as they are, were listed alongside phimosis, which unlike the other reasons at least has the advantage of sounding like a medical justification.

Phimosis and paraphimosis

Phimosis is not to be confused with paraphimosis, which is a rare condition in which the foreskin is stuck in a retracted position behind the head of the penis. Paraphimosis can cause the head of the penis to become constricted and swelling to occur. Left untreated this can become a medical emergency, with tissue death resulting from a lack of blood supply.

Circumcised males who have their entire foreskin removed obviously cannot get paraphimosis. However, the condition is rare and easily treated, so circumcision to prevent it is not warranted. Paraphimosis can be treated with manual compression and stretching, the application of substances that produce a high solute concentration to draw out water from the swollen tissue, and surgical techniques that preserve the foreskin. Circumcision is not required in most cases and should not be considered unless all these other treatment options have failed.[17]

Unlike paraphimosis, in which the foreskin is stuck in a retracted position, phimosis occurs when the foreskin fails to naturally retract by adulthood, or when the foreskin becomes non-retractable due to some other condition. Phimosis is by far the most common medical reason given for male circumcision,[18] and incredibly it is still sometimes used as a medical reason for "female circumcision".[19]

Phimosis is misdiagnosed and overdiagnosed in boys due to some doctors confusing it with the normal non-retractable foreskin during childhood.[20] Their doing so stems from an ignorance of basic anatomy, because as detailed in the previous chapter, it is perfectly normal for the foreskin to remain fused to the head of the penis until puberty. Recall also that many parents are likewise unaware that the foreskin should not be retracted until it naturally detaches from the head of the penis. The irony is that parents who forcibly retract their sons' foreskins can cause phimosis or paraphimosis, because forcible retraction can result in the formation of adhesions that cause the foreskin to abnormally fuse with the head of the penis or get stuck behind it.[21]

If men still have a tight, non-retractable foreskin as young adults, there are a number of treatment options that are less invasive than circumcision, including simple stretching techniques,[22] topical steroid creams,[23] and foreskin-sparing surgical (or plastic) correction through a procedure called a preputioplasty.[24] The use of balloon dilators might also make for a good treatment option if simple stretching techniques fail.[25] Likewise, women with phimosis have a range of treatment options that don't involve cutting off the foreskin, and it's notable that compared to males, the vast majority of doctors would never recommend such a drastic course of action for females. Topical steroids have the advantage of being non-invasive and greatly more cost effective than surgery,[26] so surgical correction is best avoided if possible. However, if other methods fail, surgery to correct phimosis is preferable to circumcision because it does not involve the removal of foreskin tissue, ensuring the foreskin and its associated functions remain. The only time circumcision is truly indicated as a treatment for phimosis is when the cause of the phimosis is a disease called lichen sclerosus, for which other treatment options have failed.

Inflammatory conditions of genitals

Lichen sclerosus[27] is a chronic inflammatory condition, the exact cause of which remains unknown, although it is thought to result from the immune system attacking the skin.[28] It is more common in females, and the most frequently affected age groups are prepubescent children, post-menopausal women, and middle-aged and elderly men.[29] Lichen sclerosus can affect the skin on any part of the body, but often involves the skin of the foreskin, anus, or vulva. In cases of lichen sclerosus involving the foreskin, the recurrent inflammation it causes can result in the buildup of scar tissue, which can restrict the foreskin, causing phimosis and the risk of paraphimosis.[30]

Circumcision is not recommended in cases of female phimosis caused by lichen sclerosus, with several surgical techniques that spare the foreskin recommended instead.[31] However, if the tissue scarring is severe enough then male circumcision is a valid treatment option for men who choose it.[32] There are, however, several treatment options that can help prevent the need for surgical intervention. Treatment with potent topical steroids can reduce inflammation and prevent damage to the foreskin tissue, with a large majority of cases of genital lichen sclerosus able to be successfully treated with topical steroids alone.[33] Other treatment options include carbon dioxide laser treatment,[34] the topical application of other drugs that suppress the immune system,[35] and steroid injections.[36]

While circumcision remains a valid treatment option for males with penile lichen sclerosus that fails to respond to other treatments, with early diagnosis and proper management, circumcision is not necessary in many cases.[37] Also, since lichen sclerosus sometimes resolves over several years and is more likely to resolve if it develops at a young age,[38] circumcision is best avoided as a treatment option in children if possible. Finally, while it is obvious that male circumcision removes lichen sclerosus of the foreskin, evidence of its benefit in treating or preventing lichen sclerosus of the head of the penis is lacking, and more than half of all men circumcised for lichen sclerosus still continue to have clinical signs of the disease, sometimes at the site of the circumcision scar, for which they require ongoing topical treatment.[39]

In addition to lichen sclerosus, there are several other inflammatory conditions that can affect the penis, including psoriasis, seborrhoeic dermatitis, lichen planus, and Zoon's balanitis. All these conditions are treatable with topical steroids or other topical medications.[40] In addition to lichen sclerosus, circumcision is sometimes also required to treat lichen planus and Zoon's balanitis, because they do not always respond to treatment with steroids or other immunosuppressive drugs. Unlike penile lichen sclerosus, however, penile lichen planus and Zoon's balanitis mostly affect middle-aged men,[41] who unlike young boys with lichen sclerosus can provide their own informed consent to circumcision as a treatment option.

Genital lichen sclerosus and lichen planus in males and females,[42] and possibly also Zoon's balanitis (which only affects males),[43] pose a risk of becoming cancerous, which may inform the decision of some men to undergo circumcision to remove foreskin tissue affected by these diseases. However, it is again noteworthy that the medical profession does not recommend cutting off parts of female genitalia affected by the same diseases *before* they have become cancerous.

Cervical cancer

The claim that male circumcision reduces cervical cancer (a cancer that affects women and transgender men) understandably seems counter-intuitive at first, but there is some logic behind it. Some argue that circumcision limits the replication and persistence of cancer-causing strains of human papillomavirus (HPV) on the penis, thereby reducing the risk of transmission to sexual partners.[44] This claim remains contentious. While circumcision does seem to reduce the persistence of HPV on the head of the penis,[45] it doesn't appear to do so on the shaft of the penis,[46] leading some to argue that the view male circumcision limits the persistence of penile HPV is the result of studies with a sampling bias in which only the head of the penis was tested.[47]

It is not necessary to get bogged down here about whether circumcision does or doesn't reduce HPV transmission, because even *if* it does, circumcision remains indefensible as an intervention strategy given that HPV vaccines are more effective, more cost-effective, and don't require the genitals of children to be mutilated.[48] A more sensible policy would be to administer the HPV vaccine to all children regardless of their sex before they reach sexual maturity. This is exactly what the Australian HPV vaccination program has done, and to great effect: even before the vaccination program, initiated in 2007, was extended to include boys in 2013, in 2011 there was an almost 40% reduction in high-grade cervical abnormalities in girls under 18 years old.[49]

Penile cancer

There is some evidence that male circumcision decreases the risk of penile cancer,[50] although this appears to be contradicted by the fact that per capita, compared to the US,[51] the incidence of penile cancer in other developed countries like Australia[52] is much lower, or in the case of the United Kingdom[53] only marginally worse, despite a significantly lower prevalence of circumcised men in these countries.[54] If circumcision really does prevent penile cancer, why does the US, where the large majority of men are circumcised, have a similar incidence of penile cancer per capita as other developed countries with proportionally fewer circumcised men? Similarly, in African countries where circumcision rates are high, rates of penile cancer remain greater than in countries with lower circumcision rates.[55] This suggests that risk factors such as poor hygiene and vaccination status are far more important than possessing a body part that might one day become cancerous.

If circumcision does reduce the risk of penile cancer, perhaps as has been argued with cervical cancer, this is due to it reducing penile HPV infection,[56] which is believed to cause roughly 40% of penile cancers. Although it has not yet been thoroughly investigated,[57] one could reasonably expect the HPV vaccine to have some benefit in reducing the incidence of penile cancer,[58] as it clearly does in reducing the incidence of cervical cancer. Again, vaccination is a preferable method of disease prevention given it doesn't involve the amputation of a body part.

Over 90% of penile cancers are a type called squamous cell carcinomas, which can develop anywhere on the penis, although most occur on the head of the penis and foreskin. The removal of the foreskin then, insofar as it removes tissue that has the potential to become cancerous, undoubtedly reduces the risk of developing such a cancer. But no doctor would recommend the routine surgical removal of the breasts or cervix in young girls to prevent breast or cervical cancer, despite cervical cancer being over six times more common,[59] and breast cancer being well over a hundred times more common,[60] not to mention more deadly, than penile cancer. Indeed, men are more likely to get breast cancer than penile cancer. The risk of developing penile cancer is so remarkably small, that less than 10 cases of penile cancer are diagnosed each year per million men in the US, accounting for less than 1% of all cancers.[61]

In addition to being rare, penile cancer mainly affects older men and has a good survival rate. That's why the circumcision of infants to prevent penile cancer makes neither practical nor economic sense. As the 2012 American Academy of Pediatrics technical report on circumcision concedes,[62] as many as 322,000 circumcisions may be required to prevent just one case of penile cancer.[63] Even on lower estimates, the number of circumcisions required remains cost prohibitive due to the cost of the procedure and its complications, compared to cost savings from cases of penile cancer prevented. Having considered all these factors, the Royal Australasian College of Physicians concluded that circumcision to protect against penile cancer is unjustified.[64]

That's certainly playing nicer than two former vice presidents of the American Cancer Society, doctors Hugh Shingleton and Clark Heath, who in 1996 wrote a letter to the American Academy of Pediatrics to "discourage" them from "promoting routine circumcision as a preventative measure for penile or cervical cancer."[65] Shingleton and Heath noted that "fatalities caused by circumcision may approximate the mortality rate from penile cancer" and concluded that "portraying routine circumcision as an effective means of prevention distracts the public from the task of avoiding the behaviors proven to contribute to penile and cervical cancer: especially cigarette smoking and unprotected sexual relations with multiple partners."[66] As Shingleton and Heath allude to, there are less invasive ways of preventing penile cancer than cutting off healthy tissue before it ever becomes cancerous, namely addressing known risk factors for the disease such as HPV infection and smoking, including through condom use, HPV vaccination, and not smoking.

It is also thought by some that phimosis is a risk factor for penile cancer because it prevents men from washing behind their foreskins and results in the buildup of smegma, and it is often asserted that smegma is associated with an increased risk of penile cancer.[67] Despite these assertions, a review of the medical literature found no firm evidence to support a link between smegma and cancer.[68] Even if it were the case that smegma can cause cancer, phimosis can almost always be treated in ways that preserve the foreskin, and once the phimosis has resolved, men can easily prevent the buildup of smegma by bathing. This last point really is the crux of the matter, because even if circumcision does reduce the risk of penile cancer by improving hygiene, men can maintain good penile hygiene by washing behind their foreskins rather than amputating them.

Clean cut?

When I was born my father wanted me circumcised because that's what was done to him, and because like many people he thought it was more hygienic. Thankfully my maternal grandfather was a doctor, and he jokingly said they might as well cut off my ears so I wouldn't have to clean behind them either. Common sense prevailed, and today I still have both my ears, and my foreskin too.

Recall that the foreskin is fused to the head of the penis until around the age of puberty, which serves to protect it. Should a baby be circumcised, there's certainly nothing hygienic about a bloody wound in a dirty diaper while it heals from surgery. Kept intact, once the foreskin eventually naturally retracts on its own, men can simply clean behind it with water.

Most men don't mind taking the extra few seconds it takes to retract their foreskin and clean behind it when bathing. Indeed, the social implications of a man not exerting the little effort it takes to keep his intact penis clean creates an incentive to do so, as it otherwise becomes difficult to maintain sexual relations with others whose standards of hygiene aren't so poor. But even without this incentive, most men are simply not that lazy. Of course, most circumcised men never get to decide whether they are circumcised, because their parents make that decision for them when they are infants or young children. Insofar as hygiene is concerned, this parental decision is seemingly made in anticipation of their son's future laziness.

While many would concede that male circumcision is unnecessary in developed countries where there is a clean water supply with which to bathe, it is often argued to be a necessary evil in developing regions that lack a clean water supply, as in some parts of Africa. I've always found this argument thoroughly unconvincing and disparaging. The insult is double edged. First, although there are parts of the developing world without a clean water supply, there are also many parts that do have clean water. Second, I fail to see how anyone can think it better to spend money on having men cut off part of their genitals because they have no clean water to wash with, rather than using that money to support non-profit organizations working to help them establish the infrastructure needed to secure a clean water supply.

Urinary tract infections

One of the most frequently touted justifications for male circumcision is that it reduces the risk of urinary tract infections (UTIs).[69] Given how often this argument is advanced you might think UTIs are the bane of every boy's existence. However, the probability of a male infant acquiring a urinary tract infection remains low, and overall UTIs are much more common in females than males,[70] yet no one is suggesting we cut off parts of girls' genitals to reduce their risk of UTIs, nor would any ethics committee ever grant permission to conduct a study to determine if doing so does in fact reduce their risk.

Often the cause of UTIs is that parents are not educated about how to bathe their newborns, and so retract their foreskins, or use soap to wash their genitals, neither of which is advisable. Forcible foreskin retraction can damage the tissue on the head of the penis and the inner foreskin, exposing it to the external environment that the previously attached foreskin was protecting it from, and creating an opening for microbes to enter. And using soap dries out the penile and vaginal mucosal lining, which makes it less acidic (in other words, more alkaline, like the soap), and kills the benign bacteria (or normal flora) that live there and normally prevent harmful (or pathogenic) bacteria from moving in. How many doctors have performed circumcisions to treat recurrent UTIs without stopping to ask parents how they bathe their baby, I wonder?

While plenty of studies suggest that UTIs are less likely to occur in circumcised males, and more likely to occur in intact males, the rates of infection in young intact males are undoubtedly overestimated due to contamination of urine samples,[71] which occurs because their foreskins cannot be retracted when collecting the samples.[72] Indeed, some have argued circumcision does not reduce the risk of UTIs, and that the apparent reduced risk of UTIs in circumcised boys is merely the result of confounding factors (like contamination) that studies have failed to control.[73] We need not get bogged down in that debate here, because even *if* male circumcision does reduce the risk of UTIs, it remains inadvisable because the benefits do not outweigh the risks,[74] it is not cost-effective,[75] and because UTIs are usually easily treated with antibiotics.[76]

In cases of recurrent UTIs, there is often an underlying anatomical abnormality of the kidneys, bladder, or the tubes connecting them that results in the backwards flow of urine (or reflux) from the bladder to the kidneys. In such cases, surgery to correct the underlying anatomical abnormality causing the reflux of urine is needed, not the removal of the foreskin, which has been shown to have no effect on the incidence of UTIs following anti-reflux surgery.[77]

Hypospadias

Hypospadias is a relatively common genital condition in which the opening of the tube that urine comes out of (the urethral opening) forms on the underside of the penis rather than on the tip of the head of the penis. While circumcision is not performed to treat hypospadias per se, often the foreskin is used in the reconstructive surgery for hypospadias, which leads to a penis that appears circumcised.[78]

Surgery for hypospadias is usually performed before 18 months of age.[79] However, as with circumcision, it has been argued by medical ethicists that most boys should not have surgery for hypospadias performed on them when they are too young to provide their own informed consent.[80] Their reasoning is the same that many apply when making the same argument about circumcision: children should be able to grow up and decide for themselves if they wish to undergo medically unnecessary surgery with the knowledge of the risks it entails.

As with circumcision, most cases of surgery for hypospadias are performed on infants in anticipation of future problems, rather than to address present problems undermining their wellbeing. Indeed, the 'problems' of hypospadias are often more social and cosmetic than functional. If the urethral opening is low enough down the shaft of the penis (proximal hypospadias), it can prevent boys from urinating while standing up and negatively affect fertility by preventing effective insemination of sperm during intercourse. But many boys with hypospadias have a urethral opening that is still located just below the head of the penis, or in the head of the penis despite not being at the very tip of it (distal hypospadias), and do not experience these functional problems. Boys with distal hypospadias are therefore more likely to reject surgery requiring circumcision for hypospadias if given the choice later in life, since the absence of functional problems means they would be trading one cosmetic problem for another, namely a slightly displaced urethral opening for a scarred penis, plus the added functional problems associated with not having a foreskin. A study of Swedish men who had surgery for hypospadias as young children found many reported the feeling of looking different due to the circumcised appearance of their penises (like most places, circumcision is not routine in Sweden).[81] Fortunately for men with distal hypospadias, techniques that preserve the foreskin can be used.[82]

Frenulum pain

The frenulum of the penis is a highly sensitive, elastic band of tissue that sits on the underside of the head of the penis, connecting it to the foreskin. Most circumcision techniques involve the destruction of the frenulum, although some have tried techniques that spare it.[83] Frenuloplasty is a surgical alternative to circumcision for the treatment of frenulum pain and scarring, which can result from an overly tight frenulum, tearing due to sexual activities, or certain inflammatory conditions. Studies of long-term outcomes and satisfaction with penile frenuloplasty as an alternative to circumcision have found that frenuloplasty is a safe alternative to circumcision, with low complication rates, high patient satisfaction, and low subsequent need or desire for circumcision.[84]

Sexually transmissible infections

A Danish study that followed more than 810,000 men over thirty-six years found that non-therapeutic circumcision in infancy or childhood does not reduce the risk of human immunodeficiency virus (HIV) or other sexually transmissible infections (STIs).[85] Indeed, the study found circumcised men had a 53% higher overall rate of STIs, with significantly higher rates of anogenital warts and syphilis observed.[86] While I'm inclined to agree with the conclusion of this study that circumcision does not reduce and may in fact increase STI transmission, research looking for possible protective effects of male circumcision against various STIs has produced mixed results.[87] That said, any doubt over whether male circumcision does or does not reduce the transmission of certain STIs is largely irrelevant, because it is beyond doubt that it does not reduce let alone eliminate the transmission risk of all of them, so a condom should still be worn.

It is a bizarre logic that trumpets circumcision of healthy, sexually immature children to reduce their risk of acquiring an infection at the age of sexual maturity, particularly when there are already proven methods of prevention that are less invasive and more cost-effective. Moreover, by the time those born recently reach sexual maturity, and become at risk of contracting STIs, there may already be new vaccines or better methods available for treating or preventing such diseases. In fact, the removal of the foreskin, and the majority of male genital mucosa along with it, could reduce the effectiveness of vaccines being developed for STIs that rely on an intact genital mucosa to work well.[88]

We've already covered the argument that circumcision might reduce the sexual transmission of cancer-causing human papillomavirus (HPV), and why it probably doesn't. We've also seen that even if it does reduce the risk of acquiring HPV, circumcision cannot be justified because there are less invasive and more cost-effective options for reducing HPV transmission, namely vaccination and condom use. Save for the option of vaccination, this same argument applies to HIV, the virus that, left untreated, is responsible for acquired immunodeficiency syndrome (AIDS). As we are about to see, the ability of circumcision to reduce HIV transmission is highly questionable.

Male circumcision and HIV "prevention"

In a letter to the *New England Journal of Medicine* in 1986, Aaron J. Fink became the first to claim that circumcision could reduce the transmission of HIV when he said, "It is my hypothesis that the presence of a foreskin predisposes both heterosexual and homosexual men to the acquisition of AIDS."[89] This was quite an outlandish assertion to be making given how little was known about HIV and AIDS at the time. In the years that followed, it became clear one of the reasons men who have sex with men are at higher risk of HIV acquisition is due to the fact HIV is much more easily transmitted by anal rather than vaginal sex.[90] Importantly, evidence clearly indicates that circumcision does *not* reduce HIV acquisition in men who have sex with men.[91] As for circumcision's impact on female-to-male HIV transmission, the argument that it provides a partial protective effect for men rests to some degree on several observational studies,[92] and to a large degree on the three randomized controlled trials (RCTs) that were conducted in South Africa,[93] Kenya[94] and Uganda.[95] Unlike the many sensationalist newspaper articles that covered the results of these RCTs, I have specifically referred to *female-to-male* transmission, because all three African RCTs showed a small reduction in HIV transmission from females to males, and only from females to males, *not* from men to women or men to men.

All three African RCTs had flawed methods and therefore questionable results. As noted by Dr. Robert Van Howe, a prominent critic of the RCTs, their nearly identical results were a consequence of identical methodologies that shared the same biases that favored the treatment effect researchers hoped for: researcher expectation bias, selection bias, participant expectation bias, lead-time bias, duration bias, attrition bias, and early termination bias.[96] Importantly, these biases alone could have provided a statistically significant difference because all three studies were what statisticians refer to as "overpowered".[97] The takeaway: the results of the RCTs should be taken with a grain of salt. Instead, they have been used as the basis of a UNAIDS campaign to circumcise millions of African boys and men. They have also been used by circumcision proponents to promote circumcision in the developed world, even though their results cannot be extrapolated beyond sub-Saharan Africa. Given the remarkable weight attributed to the RCTs by policymakers, let us consider their key problems in more detail.

All three RCTs assumed their participants to be heterosexual simply because they said they were. This assumption is naïve at best and willfully ignorant at worst. Due to the spread of extremist forms of Christianity and Islam, capital punishment has been advocated for homosexuality in sub-Saharan Africa, most notably in Uganda, where the parliamentary speaker Rebecca Kadaga chillingly referred to the "kill the gays" bill as a Christmas gift.[98] Even in South Africa (the fifth country in the world to legalize same-sex marriage) homophobia remains an ingrained cultural norm. A Pew Research Center survey conducted in 2007 found that 96% of respondents in Kenya and Uganda believed that "homosexuality should be rejected." The same was true of 64% of respondents in South Africa, where those who thought homosexuality should be accepted also dropped from 37% in 2002 to 28% in 2007.[99] (2007 was the year the Ugandan and Kenyan RCTs published their results.) It is unreasonable to expect men living in such extremely homophobic cultures would admit to having sex with other men.

The Kenyan RCT was the only one in which some men admitted to having sex with men (reportedly only 6 out of 2784 participants), and even then, all six claimed they were bisexual. Either there are no gay men in sub-Saharan Africa, or there is a problem of underreporting going on here. Aside from fear and stigma, there was another reason for gay men to lie about their sexual orientation: admitting to homosexuality would have meant exclusion from the trials, which were only concerned with a potential reduction in HIV transmission from females to males. Being ineligible to participate in the trials would have meant forgoing the financial benefits and free medical attention offered to participants.

Given we know that HIV is far more likely to be transmitted by anal sex (due to differences between vaginal and rectal tissue), the obvious question that arises is why did none of the RCTs ask about anal sex with sexual partners regardless of their participants' sexual orientation? A South African study of 310 male truck drivers found 42% admitted to having anal sex with female sex workers, and of these only 23% used a condom.[100] There is also evidence to suggest men in parts of sub-Saharan Africa who identify as heterosexual still have sex with men, and that anal sex is common there (as indeed it is everywhere).[101] Getting participants to report instances of anal sex could have avoided the problem of being unable to identify homosexual men, because the factor that's most important is the sexual behavior of participants, not their sexual orientation.

Sexual orientation is an indirect indicator of sexual behavior, and a poor one at that. Many wrongly assume that heterosexuals engage only in vaginal sex, and homosexuals in anal sex, yet there are plenty of heterosexuals who have anal sex, and plenty of homosexuals who do not. All the researchers conducting the RCTs had to do was acknowledge the fact that it's impossible to identify a high-risk group (men who have sex with men), but possible to identify a high-risk behavior (anal sex), because participants could report the latter without divulging their sexual orientation.[102] But we'll never know how the frequency of anal sex varied between groups in the RCTs, because the researchers didn't bother to ask about this important confounding factor. The failure to control for men who have sex with men, but more importantly to control for anal sex with sexual partners generally, is but one of many problems that bring into question how to interpret the results of the much-trumpeted RCTs.[103]

A major problem that plagued the RCTs was that participant dropouts were several times greater than the perceived "protective effect" of circumcision.[104] This is important, because if just some of the circumcised men who dropped out (whose HIV status therefore remained unknown) were in fact HIV-positive, results would indicate no protective effect of circumcision whatsoever. Of course, it's also unknown how many of the men who dropped out of the intact control groups became HIV-positive, but one must consider the possibility that more of the dropouts from the circumcised groups became HIV-positive than did dropouts from the intact groups. We will never know. What we do know is the men in the intact control groups had a unique motivation for dropping out – to avoid circumcision. This raises the question of why nearly equal numbers of men in the already circumcised intervention groups dropped out, and it is possible that in several cases the reason was that they were diagnosed with HIV.[105]

Incredibly, the South African RCT researchers argued that the circumcised men who dropped out wouldn't have had a great impact on results, because those who didn't attend a follow-up visit "were protected by male circumcision just as the other participants [were]."[106] Arguing from a conclusion rather than for it is poor form, and on its own is enough to indicate researcher expectation bias. But the wild speculation of the South African RCT researchers didn't stop there – they also claimed to have ruled out HIV infection in those who dropped out, arguing that the reason for the loss to follow up was due to participants moving and not their becoming HIV-positive.[107] However, if there was no follow-up, then it would have been impossible to rule out HIV infection, so for the authors to suggest it had been ruled out is misleading.

It is also important to understand that the RCTs reported *relative* rather than *absolute* values for their results. Simply put, an absolute difference is a subtraction, and a relative difference is a ratio. Whether a difference is expressed in absolute or relative terms can greatly influence how "big" that difference appears. For example, say the risk of relapse during a five-year period following cancer remission is 10 in 100 (10%) in patients treated with one treatment regimen, and 5 in 100 (5%) in patients treated with a second treatment regimen. If this is expressed as an absolute difference, the second treatment regimen reduces the five-year risk of relapse by 5%.[108] Expressed as a relative difference, however, the second treatment regimen reduces the risk of relapse by 50% compared to the first treatment regimen.[109] These numbers are both saying the same thing, but clearly the result expressed as a relative difference sounds more impressive.

For simplicity, if we combine the three African female-to-male RCTs, a total of 5,411 men were circumcised and 5,497 were intact controls. Of these men, 64 (1.18%) circumcised and 137 (2.49%) intact men became HIV-positive, resulting in an absolute difference of just 1.31%;[110] a result which doesn't sound nearly as impressive as the widely reported relative 60% protective effect, and which could easily be reduced to nothing if only a fraction of men who dropped out from the circumcised intervention groups were in fact HIV-positive.

Perhaps cutting away the mucosal tissue of young girls' genitals could reduce HIV transmission. We'll never know, because thankfully no ethics committee would ever permit researchers to cut off healthy female genitalia to find out. The fact also remains that results from trials of adult, sexually active, reportedly heterosexual African males cannot be applied to sexually immature children, let alone extrapolated to dictate health policy in the developed world, where the main groups affected by HIV are men or transgender women who have sex with men and injecting drug users, not heterosexual men. Indeed, a study of almost 570,000 men in Ontario, Canada, found that circumcision was not associated with the risk of men acquiring HIV;[111] a result that may well have been replicated by the African RCTs had they not suffered from biases and flawed methods.

Of enormous concern is how despite their many flaws and limitations, major policy decisions have been made based on the African RCT results. In 2011, UNAIDS released its *Joint strategic action framework to accelerate the scale-up of voluntary medical male circumcision for HIV prevention in Eastern and Southern Africa: 2012–2016* (hereafter the UNAIDS report). The UNAIDS report called for the "voluntary" mass circumcision of boys and men in Eastern and Southern Africa and laid out a two-stage process to achieve this.[112] In the first "catch-up" phase, it advocates for the voluntary circumcision of adult males, and in the second "sustainability" phase, it advocates for routine circumcision of infants. This seems to contradict its initial ethos, given that circumcision of children too young to consent is always involuntary. The UNAIDS report also ignored the fact that the indiscriminate circumcision of all boys includes boys who will grow up to be gay, and for whom circumcision would provide no claimed protection against HIV transmission at all, which doesn't seem very fair to them.

Reading the UNAIDS report, I was struck by a line in which UNAIDS absolves itself from all responsibility for its plan to circumcise tens of millions of boys and men in Africa, stating in the fine print of their report that: "UNAIDS does not warrant that the information published in this publication is complete and correct and shall not be liable for any damages incurred as a result of its use." Talk about suspect. If I was advocating spending billions of dollars on the involuntary circumcision of millions of baby boys, and the "voluntary" circumcision of millions more men whose health literacy in many cases is poor, I'd want to be certain my information was correct before proposing such a drastic course of action, wouldn't you? I'd want to be sure my recommendations were based on mountains of mutually supportive medical evidence, and not just a few poorly conducted randomized control trials, especially when those recommendations run counter to peak organizations of medical doctors all around the world, none of which recommend routine infant circumcision as a preventative health measure. Were the authors of the UNAIDS report even medical doctors or researchers? None of the authors of the UNAIDS report put their name to it, and my multiple requests for the authors' names and credentials have gone unanswered.

The authors' names weren't the only thing missing from the UNAIDS report. Also missing was reference to a fourth African RCT conducted in Uganda, which looked at the impact of circumcision on HIV transmission from *males to females*. You probably haven't heard of it, though, because unlike the three female-to-male trials, its results weren't widely reported by the media. This was perhaps because it found a relative 61% *increase* in HIV transmission from circumcised men to women, causing the trial to be terminated early.[113]

As groups that take the results of the African RCTs seriously, it is surprising that the WHO and UNAIDS are promoting a campaign of mass male circumcision based on claims it results in a relative 60% reduction of female-to-male HIV transmission, despite claims it also results in a relative 60% *increase* in male-to-female HIV transmission. This fact alone should have been enough to give one pause before recommending a campaign of mass circumcision in HIV endemic regions, but the trial's researchers remained undeterred. Despite the complete lack of benefit to men who are already HIV positive, the lack of evidence that male circumcision reduces the risk of HIV transmission from men to women, and indeed their own evidence indicating it increased the risk of HIV transmission to women, the researchers of the male-to-female RCT nonetheless concluded it advisable for HIV positive men to be circumcised.[114] This recommendation is reckless and irresponsible in the extreme.

Circumcised men who have unprotected sex remain at much greater risk of acquiring HIV and other STIs than intact men who wear a condom. So, you may well ask, what is the point of circumcising men if they still need to wear a condom or take other precautions? It could be argued that their being circumcised might help reduce their risk were a condom to break, or that no matter what there will always be some men who have condomless sex, so it's better they at least have some protection through circumcision. Again, I don't think circumcision offers them any such protection, but even if it did, the 1.31% absolute reduction in risk is trivial. It would be far better for HIV-negative people who have condomless sex to take HIV pre-exposure prophylaxis (or PrEP) tablets, given PrEP reduces the risk of HIV acquisition by more than 99%.[115] It would also be far better for people to take post-exposure prophylaxis (or PEP) for HIV should a condom break during sex. Finally, it is worth noting that adults who choose to have unprotected sex do so at their own risk, and that many men who choose to have protected sex were circumcised as sexually immature children too young to consent on the presumption they wouldn't.

The African RCTs were conducted well over a decade ago, and in addition to the proven efficacy of PrEP, it has since been established that people living with HIV cannot sexually transmit the virus, even if they have condomless sex, so long as they are on treatment and have a sustained undetectable viral load.[116] This incredible finding is the basis of the Undetectable = Untransmittable (or U=U) campaign. Investing in widespread availability of PrEP and condoms, and ensuring people living with HIV have access to affordable treatment and medical care so they can remain undetectable and therefore unable to sexually transmit HIV, are far superior options for preventing new HIV transmissions compared to circumcision, because they are proven to work, and because they don't involve mutilating people.

In short, even *if* the removal of the foreskin really does reduce the risk of men acquiring HIV from vaginal sex, the risk reduction is trivial, it provides absolutely no protection to women or men who have sex with men, and as detailed earlier, either limited or no protection against other STIs. In other words, preventative measures such as PrEP and condoms still need to be used. This last point is particularly important, because it is possible circumcised men may be less likely to use a condom given that their penises are desensitized as a result, or if they are under the impression their circumcised status provides them adequate protection, as media reports in Africa indicate many men are.[117]

We have already seen troubling signs of the voluntary male medical circumcision (VMMC) initiative reducing condom use in a study of circumcised South African high-school males.[118] I believe the flippant attitude toward condom use following circumcision results from the misconception that circumcision *prevents* HIV transmission. Circumcision does not prevent HIV transmission. At best it slightly *reduces the risk* of HIV transmission, and in so doing prevents some new HIV infections. That's an important distinction, because to "prevent transmission" carries connotations of complete protection, whereas "reduce the risk of transmission" does not.

History might not repeat, but it rhymes, and a similar debate has been had before. As the late medical historian Robert Darby observed, there's a noticeable similarity between nineteenth-century claims circumcision "prevented" transmission of syphilis and the modern-day claims circumcision "prevents" transmission of HIV, or as Darby put it, "In each case, a rather slender and over-worked body of evidence became the justification for a towering clinical edifice (and in the case of Africa, a giant, foreign-funded, job-generating service industry) that soon began to look too heavy for its foundations."[119] It is little wonder that those promoting the mass circumcision of African boys and men have been accused of cultural imperialism.[120]

. . .

I began this book by saying that of all the arguments for routine circumcision of infant boys, the argument from medical benefits was the only one that stood a chance as a potential justification for the practice. Having now reviewed all the potential medical benefits of male circumcision, I trust readers will agree they are negligible, if not non-existent, depending on the specific claim in question. But even if readers disagree, and still accept the medical claims of circumcision proponents in part or in full, it remains necessary to also consider the complications of circumcision, because as with any surgery, one must not just consider the potential benefits, but also weigh them against the risks.

4

A bloody mess

This was a hard chapter to write, and no doubt will be a hard chapter to read, especially for circumcised men. Take a moment to consider your headspace before reading on, and feel free to skip ahead to the next chapter if needed.

Surgeons use several different techniques to circumcise infant boys, but whatever the procedure, it always begins by restraining the baby. Nowadays, after being strapped down, the baby likely receives a pain-relieving injection (or local anesthetic), as well as a numbing gel applied to the penile skin (or topical anesthetic), and often also oral sugar solutions, although the ability of sugar to provide pain relief is highly questionable.[1] The use of pain relievers for circumcision is, however, a relatively recent phenomenon. The lack of pain relief historically available to infants was not limited to backyard procedures performed by the medically unqualified. Indeed, even as late as the 1990s, most circumcisions performed by doctors in North America were performed without anesthetic.[2]

The shift toward using pain relief for circumcisions may be considered progress of a kind. However, even when used, topical anesthetic probably has little effect, as it's unable to penetrate the dorsal penile nerves, which are located under a layer of connective tissue beneath the skin.[3] It's also common for babies to wet themselves, washing off some of the topical anesthetic, rendering it even less effective, if indeed it has any tangible effect at all. Unfortunately, the local anesthetic injections aren't much better. The injections themselves would be quite painful, and several are required to properly numb the area. There is also a risk of hitting the dorsal penile artery to reach the dorsal penile nerve, or the urethra (the tube urine comes out of) to reach the ventral nerve branches. Oddly, parents often worry their baby boy is too young and delicate to receive an anesthetic injection yet show an apparent lack of concern over him having the most sensitive part of his penis cut off.

With the baby restrained, and – if he is lucky – numb to at least some of the pain he is about to endure, he is then most likely subjected to one of either the Gomco, Mogen, or Plastibell surgical techniques.[4]

The Gomco technique (Figure 1) uses the Gomco clamp, developed in 1935 by New York doctors Hiram Yellen and Aaron Goldstein.[5] Similar clamps designed to crush the skin, which reduce bleeding and the need for sutures, have been developed, but none have ever proved as popular as the Gomco clamp. The Gomco technique begins with the insertion of a metal probe or closed forceps under the foreskin to forcibly separate the fused foreskin from the head of the penis (Figure 1A). The foreskin is then peeled back behind the overhanging rim (or coronal sulcus) at the base of the head of the penis. If the foreskin cannot be pulled back behind the head of the penis, then forceps are used to crush the foreskin lengthways, which becomes the line down which an incision (or dorsal slit) is made so the foreskin can be pulled back further (Figure 1B). A metal device with a bell-shaped end is then placed over the head of the penis (Figure 1C), and using forceps, the foreskin is pulled over it and tied tightly with string (Figure 1D). A metal clamp is then connected to the bell-shaped covering, and the foreskin is cut off at the base of the clamp using a scalpel (Figure 1E).

Figure 1 – Gomco technique

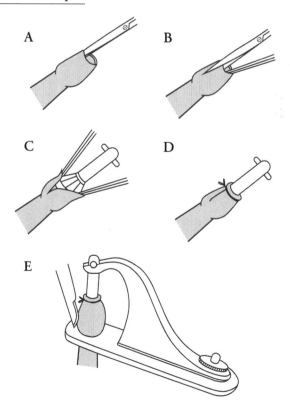

A

B

C

D

E

The Mogen technique (Figure 2) uses the Mogen clamp, developed in 1955 by another New Yorker, Rabbi Harry Bronstein.[6] This technique is commonly used by mohels who perform Jewish ritual circumcisions, but is also used by some doctors. It too begins with the forced separation of the fused mucosa of the inner foreskin and head of the penis (Figure 2A). This is followed by the foreskin being lifted over the head of the penis and placed between the open jaws of the Mogen clamp (Figure 2B), which is then closed for a few minutes to crush the foreskin to help prevent bleeding (Figure 2C), before the foreskin is cut off after the point the clamp has crushed it (Figure 2D). The clamp is then opened, and downward pressure is applied on the penile skin to push it back behind the head of the penis.

Figure 2 – Mogen technique

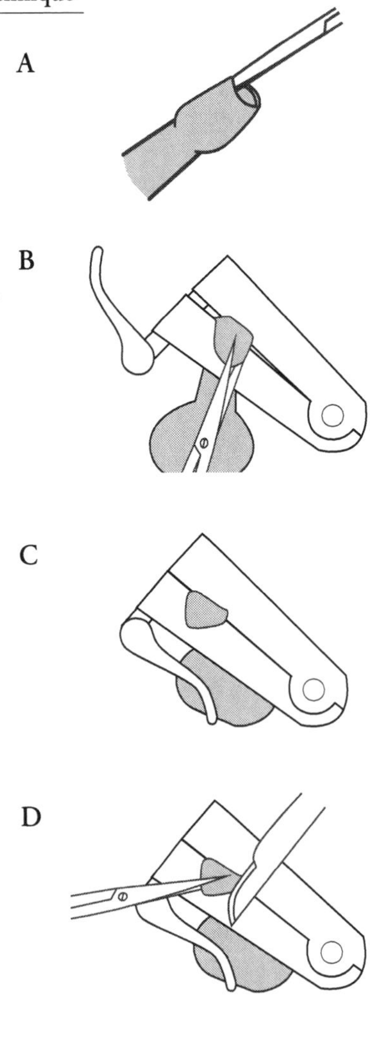

The Plastibell technique uses the Plastibell, developed by the Hollister Company in the 1950s. The Plastibell technique also begins with the forced separation of the fused mucosa of the inner foreskin and head of the penis (Figure 3A). This is followed by a dorsal slit of the foreskin (Figure 3B). The foreskin is then peeled back behind the head of the penis, and a plastic device with a bell-shaped end (the Plastibell) is placed over the head of the penis (Figure 3C). Using forceps, the foreskin is then pulled over it and tied tightly with string (Figure 3D), before being cut off with a surgical knife or scissors just after the point where it is tied (Figure 3E). The handle of the bell-shaped plastic device is then snapped off, leaving just the bell and the tied penile skin in place (Figure 3F). The skin tissue remaining after the point at which the skin is tied dies and separates from the bell several days later.

Figure 3 – Plastibell technique

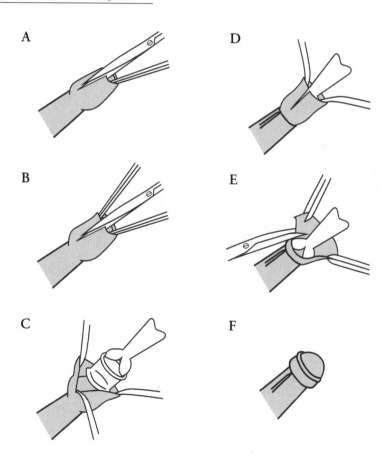

While the Gomco, Plastibell and Mogen techniques are the most popular, they are by no means the only techniques used by surgeons to circumcise boys, with other devices and "free-hand" techniques also used. The surgical techniques used to perform circumcisions, and the precise nature of their execution, vary depending on where and by whom the circumcisions are performed. It must also be said that globally, many circumcisions are performed neither by a surgeon nor with sterile equipment. Often male circumcision consists of (usually male) relatives holding the boy down while one of them cuts the foreskin off with a sharp knife or scissors, which might have been cleaned with boiling water first. (Surgical equipment is properly sterilized by very high pressure and temperature in a machine called an autoclave.) Whatever the nature of the operation, whoever performs it, and at whatever age, in all cases the circumcision procedure remains exactly as it sounds – painful.

I've done my best to describe the most common circumcision procedures, but nothing compares to watching them. A simple search for "circumcision" on YouTube reveals many horrifying videos, and it appears that consent to use the footage of the operation, like the consent to perform it, was never sought from the boys who were cut.

Parents considering circumcising their sons ought to watch several videos of circumcisions being performed, so they know exactly what they're planning to put their boys through. It's important to watch the whole procedure from start to finish, to listen to the screams of those for whom the anesthetic clearly didn't work, or who didn't receive any, and to remember that those who are silent are likely in a state of shock. Once you have watched such videos, remember that what remains unseen are the many complications that can arise following circumcision; complications that will now be examined.

In discussing these complications, I will refer to them as either common or rare, rather than provide specific statistics for the rate of complications. I do this because complication rates are subject to change and vary regionally according to the skills of the surgeons or people performing circumcisions. For example, researchers in Nigeria concluded that they could bring down their "unacceptably high" overall circumcision complication rate of 20.2% by training circumcision practitioners.[7] There's a thought. A better one would be to not perform unnecessary circumcisions in the first place.

Blood loss

Perhaps the most obvious complication that can arise from a procedure involving the excision of tissue is blood loss, and indeed it is one of the more common complications of circumcision. This can present a serious problem for children born with bleeding disorders such a hemophilia, in which their blood cannot clot properly. Despite the availability of prenatal diagnostic tests for hemophilia, many newborns are still only diagnosed after a bleeding episode. A study found that 30% of hemophilia diagnoses in newborn British boys occurred following circumcision bleeds.[8] However, most of these boys were cut before 1970, so with circumcision now rare in the UK, and the use of fibrin glue during circumcisions to control bleeding having become standard, it is now less common for bleeding disorders to be diagnosed following circumcision-related bleeding in the UK.

Fibrin glue is derived from human blood plasma, so it carries the small risk of transmitting viral infections like hepatitis C, and it can sometimes also trigger adverse and allergic reactions.[9] For this reason, instead of using fibrin glue to control bleeding, some doctors use injections of clotting factors not derived from human plasma to help prevent bleeding from occurring in the first place.[10] Some use neither or both. However, clotting factors do not always successfully prevent bleeding complications.[11] Moreover, their use in the first place depends both on the doctor knowing that the baby has a bleeding disorder prior to the circumcision, which many don't, and on established protocols that require their use, which do not exist in many places. For example, a 2015 survey of pediatric hematologists at hemophilia treatment centers in the US found that 78% did not have established protocols for the management of circumcision of newborns with hemophilia.[12] Whatever way those with bleeding disorders are managed, the problem with newborns losing blood is they cannot afford to lose very much of it.

Infection

The circumcision wound doesn't just let blood out, it can also let microbes in, which is a problem in an era of disease-causing bacteria that are resistant to most antibiotics in our arsenal. One such type of bacteria is *Staphylococcus aureus*, which has a strain resistant to the antibiotic methicillin (MRSA) now endemic in hospitals. The spread of MRSA has serious consequences for everyone, including newborns.

One study of newborn babies found the mortality rate of those with MRSA was 24.6%.[13] The study also found a mortality rate of 39% even in cases of methicillin-sensitive staph infection (MSSA) if the onset of infection was within 48 hours of delivery, compared to 7.3% if it was more than 2 days after delivery.[14] This is concerning, because circumcision increases the risk of infection, including staphylococcal infection;[15] and because in the US most newborn circumcisions are performed within the first couple days after birth, before the baby even leaves the hospital.[16] MRSA and MSSA infections following circumcision are rare, but given such high mortality rates, particularly when there is early onset of infection, how can any doctor justify performing circumcisions on newborns in the first few days after birth?

The fact that MRSA is common in hospitals might lead some to argue it's better to perform circumcisions in community clinics. However, the overall complication rate in the community remains higher,[17] and MRSA has also been a problem in the community since the late 1990s. The less severe MSSA is also increasingly displaced by community-associated MRSA, which is more virulent and resistant to antibiotics.[18] MRSA is by no means the only bacteria that can cause infection, and along with other types of bacteria, MRSA can cause a flesh-eating infection (or necrotizing fasciitis), in which dead tissue needs to be surgically removed,[19] causing disfigurement.

The problem of antimicrobial resistance is quite literally evolving, and public health authorities around the world are watching on nervously, but the emergence of antibiotic-resistant microbes and the risk of infection with them following medically unnecessary neonatal circumcision is far too often overlooked.

Scarring

Many circumcised men are not aware of it,[20] but all of them have a circumcision scar that encircles the penis at the point the foreskin was cut off. In addition to this scar, circumcision can also sometimes result in keloid scars, which form because of abnormal wound healing that causes excessive collagen build up in the skin at the site of injury.

The tendency toward abnormal wound healing exists in certain people prior to any injury, and it is unfortunate that many discover they are prone to keloid formation after circumcision, because for many it is the first wound that they experience in their lives. Treatment of keloid scars involves steroid creams and injections, as well as surgical excision, although the recurrence of keloid scars following surgical removal is common.[21]

Buried penis

A buried (or concealed or trapped) penis is a rare complication of circumcision that results from overzealous removal of the penile skin, coupled with plump skin surrounding the penis such that the penis is buried beneath mounds of fat, with healing occurring within the fat pad.[22] In cases of buried penis the untrained eye could be forgiven for thinking the penis had been amputated, with worried parents sometimes reporting that their sons' penises seem to have disappeared after their circumcision.[23]

Buried penis may require surgery if it does not spontaneously resolve as the infant gets older.[24] Sometimes boys are born with a buried penis, in which case circumcision is definitely inadvisable, as it will only worsen the condition.[25]

Penile adhesions

Penile adhesions are a relatively common complication of circumcision, not to be confused with the normal adhesion of the inner foreskin to the head of the penis that naturally detaches over time. Following circumcision, penile adhesions can occur between the shaft skin and the head of the penis as the wounded tissue around the shaft skin heals itself.

Penile adhesions can be manually separated, and often spontaneously resolve with time, whereas skin bridges are more extensive, thicker adhesions that often require surgical intervention.[26] Left uncorrected, skin bridges can tether the penis during erection, causing deformity and pain.[27]

Urethral fistula

Circumcision can sometimes result in single or multiple holes in the penis where there shouldn't be any. When these holes connect with the urethra, they are referred to as urethral fistulas. This rare complication of circumcision can result from suturing to control bleeding or injury to the urethra caused by surgical clamps.[28] As you would expect, urethral fistulas result in multiple streams of urine during urination.

Meatal stenosis

Meatal stenosis is the narrowing of the opening of the urethra.[29] It occurs almost exclusively in circumcised boys and is one of the most common complications of circumcision, however, the condition is underreported due to the lack of long-term follow-up after circumcision.[30] Meatal stenosis often results in pain during urination and a narrow, high-velocity stream of urine.[31]

Kidney failure

Kidney failure can occur following urinary obstruction and urine retention, which is a rare but serious complication of circumcisions performed with the Plastibell.[32] The retention of urine leads to subsequent rupture of the bladder and life-threatening kidney failure.[33] Kidney failure can also occur because of urinary obstruction caused by overzealous bandaging or by swelling following circumcision.[34]

Penile disfigurement and amputation

In 2017, a Swiss doctor was acquitted for accidentally cutting off a four-year-old boy's penis during his circumcision.[35] The accident happened because the doctor let the boy's father sit in on his son's circumcision to take photographs. The son turned to his father as he was about to take a picture, turning his hips as he turned the rest of his body, at which point the doctor accidentally cut off the boy's penis. What's wrong with this picture? It is tempting to say everything: the mutilation of one's child is not a moment for the family photo album; non-consensual, medically unnecessary genital cutting is not medicine; and child mutilators, even those with medical degrees, should be punished, not protected by the law. This case is by no means the only recent case of penile amputation, with many others being reported by the media.[36] Many more are never reported due to non-disclosure clauses in settlement contracts with doctors.

Poorly timed photographs are of course not a common cause of penile disfigurement or amputation, which typically occurs because of poor surgical execution. For example, the use of a metal bell during the Gomco technique that is too small to properly cover the head of the penis can lead to accidental incision of the head of the penis, while the use of one that is too large always results in the removal of too much penile skin,[37] which can cause painful and shortened erections. Circumcision can also result in curvature of the penis,[38] which some may consider a form of disfigurement. The use of a Plastibell that is too small can likewise result in disfigurement, because the pressure of the small bell on the head of the penis can cause the tissue to die (this is known as pressure necrosis).[39]

Gangrene

Gangrene is a type of tissue death (or necrosis) caused by insufficient blood supply. It is a rare but particularly devastating complication of circumcision, which can occur because of tight bandaging following circumcision creating a tourniquet effect, or from the inappropriate use during circumcision of a particular type of electrosurgery, called monopolar diathermy, which can cause blood to clot at the base of penis.[40]

Methemoglobinemia

In rare cases topical and local anesthetics used for circumcision have been reported to cause a potentially life-threatening condition called methemoglobinemia.[41] Infants less than three months of age are more susceptible to this condition, in which the oxygen-carrying hemoglobin of red blood cells is oxidized to become methemoglobin, which has less oxygen-carrying capacity.[42] As the level of methemoglobin in the blood increases it becomes more and more noticeable, because the baby's cells are being progressively starved of oxygen, turning the baby pale blue. If the amount of methemoglobin reaches high enough levels it can result in death.

Death

It's difficult to determine exactly how many deaths result from circumcision complications, but we know they happen. The reason it's difficult to attribute deaths to complications associated with circumcision is because such information is often not reported on death certificates. For example, the death certificate may only list infection entering the bloodstream (or septicemia) as the cause of death, when in fact the infection occurred as a complication of circumcision. Such difficulties aside, a 2010 study estimated that approximately 117 male infants die every year in the US because of circumcision complications, accounting for 1.3% of all deaths in male newborns.[43]

Psychological trauma

Circumcision proponents often argue that one of the benefits of circumcising infants is that they are too young to remember the pain of being circumcised. This is an excuse without excuse. The fact someone cannot remember being harmed is not a justification for harming them. Just as it's not okay to abuse someone who is unconscious or who has Alzheimer's, it's not okay to abuse children too young to remember it. If anything, harming those who can't remember is worse than harming those who can, because at least those who can remember the harm done to them are better able to seek justice for being wronged. The notion that infants forget the pain of circumcision is not only a horrible excuse for a practice that is ethically wrong, mounting evidence suggests that it is factually wrong too.

A Canadian study found that circumcised infants showed a greater response to pain than intact infants during subsequent routine vaccination, and that of the circumcised infants, those who received anesthetic prior to their procedure showed a reduced pain response compared to those who did not.[44] Some have argued that the hypersensitivity to pain that circumcised children display is suggestive of post-traumatic stress disorder (PTSD).[45] Indeed, other studies have found evidence of PTSD in circumcised boys,[46] and suggested that circumcision can have a lasting negative impact on many men's body image and self-esteem. Few would question the same results found in girls who have been subjected to female genital mutilation,[47] and there is no reason to think, as far as the psychology of physical trauma is concerned, that what is true for girls and women is not also true for boys and men.

While psychiatry is a particularly complicated field of medicine, there is enough evidence to suggest infants do, on some level and for some time, remember the circumcision pain they suffered. What's more, many boys around the world are circumcised when they are clearly old enough to remember it, and those who don't remember it may be suffering post-traumatic amnesia.[48]

Even if men have no memory of ever being circumcised, the knowledge of what was done to them is enough to cause psychological harm. Every time I have spoken publicly about circumcision, I have seen men in the audience break down in tears. For many men, the impact of learning that they were circumcised, and the knowledge of the harm that was done to them, causes them to suffer feelings of anger, loss, shame, violation, fear, distrust, and even envy of intact men.[49] Increasingly, many men are turning to foreskin restoration as a way of addressing these feelings, and of regaining some of what was taken from them.

Foreskin restoration

Some may disagree with circumcision being described as an irreversible procedure, given that hundreds of thousands of men have already restored or are currently restoring their foreskins. However, as an understanding of the anatomy of the foreskin that was removed makes clear, while it is certainly possible to achieve something with the superficial appearance of a foreskin, and even to restore some of its functions, circumcision remains irreversible in the sense that circumcised men can never fully regain the foreskin tissue they were born with and all its associated functions. For example, an important part of the foreskin that cannot be restored is the ridged band, which is a highly sensitive piece of tissue that encircles the tip of the foreskin and helps to keep the glans covered by the foreskin. The inability to reproduce the ridged band during the restoration process can sometimes result in an overly loose foreskin that does not properly cover the head of the penis. It is also not possible to replace the foreskin's many nerve endings and sensory receptors, or the mucosal tissue of the inner foreskin that was removed by circumcision. None of this means that foreskin restoration is not worthwhile, as many men who have restored their foreskins report improved sensation and pleasure;[50] it only means that these men will never be able to regain an anatomically complete foreskin and the full level of sexual and protective functions it provides.

The most common restoration technique is non-surgical and utilizes weights to apply tension to the shaft of the penis, so that over time the skin grows to cover the head of the penis and resemble a foreskin. The downside of this method, often referred to as "tugging", is that it requires consistent tension being applied over a long period. It's also not without risk, as there is the possibility of further damaging tissue from the use of excessive force.

Surgical foreskin restoration methods achieve faster results but remain uncommon due to their being much more expensive and carrying a much greater risk of complications. Another deterrent is that restorative surgery involves the grafting of skin onto the penis, skin that is usually acquired from the scrotum. One such procedure described has multiple stages, and requires the scrotum being wrapped around the penis for several months.[51]

That so many men go to such lengths to restore their foreskins stands as testament to the fact many are unhappy with the choice that was made for them when they were circumcised at the behest of their parents. Any expecting parent considering circumcising their son should consider that their son might one day choose to endure uncomfortable, costly, and arduous restoration procedures because of their decision. Indeed, the number of men engaging in foreskin restoration is increasing. TLC Tugger is an American-based company that produces several products that assist with foreskin restoration. It is struggling to keep up with demand. As further evidence of a growing foreskin restoration movement, support groups like the National Organization of Restoring Men (NORM) have established branches in many countries. For men wanting to learn more about foreskin restoration, NORM offers advice and provides a list of people who can be contacted for foreskin restoration tips on its website. For those interested in foreskin restoration, I also recommend reading *The Joy of Uncircumicising* by Jim Bigelow.

...

The next chapter will deal with the arguments of those who find circumcised penises more aesthetically pleasing, but whatever your thoughts about the end result, there's nothing pretty about the circumcision procedure itself. Circumcision is a bloody mess forced on boys who will forever have to live with what was done to them, excluding of course those who die because of it.

5

A view to a cut

If you've ever seen ancient Greek male statues you've probably noticed they tend to have one small thing in common – they aren't terribly well endowed. It turns out the reason for this is not just that these men modeled nude before central heating existed. As the art historian Kenneth Dover wrote in *Greek Homosexuality*, the visual arts show us the aesthetic criteria by which the ancient Greeks judged male genitals.[1] In his study of vase paintings, Dover notes that the typical penis of a young man, whether human or divine, is depicted as thin and short, often with a foreskin that "is so long that the end of the glans is hardly more than halfway from the base of the penis to the tip of the foreskin."[2] The reason for this, according to another art historian, Ellen Oredsson, is that "all representations of large penises in ancient Greek art and literature are associated with foolish, lustful men, or the animal-like satyrs."[3] This stood in contrast to the ideal Greek man, who "was rational, intellectual and authoritative. He may still have had a lot of sex, but this was unrelated to his penis size, and his small penis allowed him to remain coolly logical."[4]

Although a prominent foreskin was considered desirable by most ancient Greek and Roman men, it was particularly important to athletes who competed in the nude, whose *beau ideal* of a Hellenistic athlete was one with a foreskin that fully covered the glans. Perhaps these athletes would have been as embarrassed competing with a short foreskin then as most would be competing nude today. For men with a short foreskin the first century writer Aulus Cornelius Celsus details a procedure in his *De medicina*, in which a circular cut was made at the base of the shaft of the penis, so the skin could be pulled forward to achieve the desired length. For men who had been circumcised, a more radical operation is described, in which a circular cut was made around the base of the head of the penis (or corona), and the shaft skin "degloved" from the underlying tissue, allowing it to be pulled over the head of the penis, with plaster packed between the skin and the glans to prevent adhesions forming between the two.[5]

Clearly standards of beauty change, and that includes standards of beauty concerning genitalia. Though the ancient Greeks would not have approved, today it seems that larger penises are in vogue just about everywhere, as are circumcised penises in some places. The fact is some people think genitals that are surgically altered to look a particular way look better than they do in their natural state. It is a belief they use to justify the genital cutting of themselves or, far more often, of children too young to share their belief or defend themselves. In the developed world, this argument from aesthetics is often applied to boys and men as a justification for male circumcision, and it is increasingly being applied to adult women for cosmetic genital surgery. Indeed, male circumcision is so common in some places, and yet so rarely discussed, that I've met circumcised men who thought their penises were that way when they were born. Doctors know better of course, yet many in America have never even seen an intact penis, because most of the male population there is cut, and depictions of male anatomy in American medical textbooks often only contain images of circumcised penises.[6]

Thankfully, the view that mutilated female genitals look better is not as widespread as it is for males, but worryingly it's a view that's gaining ground in several developed countries, with cosmetic female genital surgery on the rise. The reason why, according to plastic surgeons, is that women want to improve their self-esteem (society teaches them to be ashamed of the way their genitals look), and because they want to be more attractive to men (who they are afraid will find their genitals unappealing). Among these surgeries are clitoral hood reduction (otherwise known as Type I female genital mutilation), and labiaplasty (otherwise known as Type II female genital mutilation).

The clitoral hood is the female foreskin, a similar (or homologous) structure to the male foreskin. Labiaplasty is the surgical reduction of the inner and outer labia (the flaps of tissue that surround the vulva). In Australia, the increasing number of women seeking to have their labia reduced has in part been fueled by prudish pornography classification rules, which require the digital alteration of images of vaginas so that labia can't be seen.[7] This is not limited to Australia, however, with the porn industry having long infantilised women's genitalia. It appears many men are now under the impression labia don't exist, and this has left many women wishing theirs didn't.

Despite adult women going under the knife with increasing frequency in the hopes of improving their appearance – an act that has more recently begun to include genital alteration – as far as I am aware people in the developed world have yet to argue (as many do with boys) that young girls should involuntarily undergo genital surgery to improve their appearance. But if there comes a time when most women have surgically altered genitals, thereby normalizing that appearance, in the same way that male circumcision has become normalized, we should expect that there would be strong support for the surgical alteration of young girls' genitals. We must remain vigilant if we are to avoid this violation of young girls' bodies and rights.

Male circumcision remains much more common in the developed world than the surgical alteration of female genitalia. In the US alone, well over a million newborn boys are circumcised every year,[8] whereas, for example, only 10,774 women had a labiaplasty in 2016.[9] Aside from the dramatic difference in those totals, the notable difference between the two is that male circumcision is most often performed on boys without their consent, whereas female genital cutting – again I stress only in the US and the rest of the developed world – is mostly performed on adult women who have provided their informed consent before going under the knife.[10] The notable similarity in both cases is that the genital alteration appears to be performed largely for the appeasement of men, and is fueled by the medical–industrial complex, particularly in the US.

Paging Dr. Malpractice

As with male genital cutting, the push promoting female cutting in the US has, incredibly, come from its medical community, which has a sordid history of promoting unnecessary surgeries and pathologizing healthy body parts in the quest for profits. Indeed, "cosmetic surgery" is an oxymoron, because "surgery" implies the operation is for the treatment of some injury or disorder, although I'll continue to use the term for ease of reading.

By the 1980s, only a couple of decades after the first breast implant, as many as a million women in the US had undergone breast augmentation.[11] The vast majority of these breast enlargements were done for cosmetic rather than reconstructive purposes, and there would be millions more where that came from if the American Society for Plastic and Reconstructive Surgeons (ASPRS) had anything to say about it. In 1982, in response to a decision by the Food and Drug Administration to put breast implants in a stricter regulatory category due to safety concerns, ASPRS swiftly submitted a public comment in which they claimed small breasts were physical deformities in need of correction to prevent feelings of inadequacy and low self-confidence due to a lack of perceived femininity.[12]

Almost as ridiculous as the ASPRS statement was the $4 million it spent on a marketing campaign a year later that claimed women with small breasts had a newly coined disease called "micromastia". The advertisements promised women breasts that looked more "normal" and "natural" after enlargement.[13] With statements like that (coming from medical professionals no less) you can see how some women with smaller breasts at the time might have suffered from low self-esteem and feelings of inadequacy. And *not* as luck would have it, but as a group of conniving doctors unworthy of the profession would have it, the very doctors who shamed women into feelings of inadequacy had an expensive solution to make them feel better about themselves.

Today, with hundreds of thousands of American women having their breasts enlarged every year,[14] and the plastic surgery industry generating more than $18 billion a year in the US,[15] it's fitting that the American Society of Plastic and Reconstructive Surgeons changed its name in 1999 to simply be the American Society of Plastic Surgeons.[16] Of course, reconstructive surgeries are still performed, but they pale in comparison to cosmetic surgeries, with 17.7 million cosmetic procedures, compared to 5.8 million reconstructive procedures in the US in 2018.[17] The result is not only that wait times for reconstructive breast surgery are significantly longer than wait times for cosmetic breast surgery;[18] but that many people suffer for months or even years waiting to have, for example, hip or knee surgery, because many talented doctors who would make fine orthopedic surgeons instead train as plastic surgeons to cash in on vanity instead of healing the sick.

While we should continue to affirm the right of adults to consent to cosmetic surgeries, this doesn't mean we should ignore the fact that a multi-billion-dollar industry has been built around convincing healthy people they should feel insecure because they don't look a certain way, and that they need unnecessary cosmetic surgery to be happy or complete. Call that what you want, but it certainly isn't medicine.

The price of vanity

Male circumcision is regularly undertaken as a purely cosmetic procedure, and like most cosmetic procedures it doesn't come cheap. The Circumcision Center in Atlanta, Georgia, which only circumcises adults, charges upwards of $2,500 (USD) for first-time circumcisions, which only take 90 minutes, of which 30 minutes is spent in consultation with the doctor. For those not happy with the cosmetic appearance after their circumcision, revisions can be performed for another $2,500.[19] On the cheaper end of the scale, the California-based company Gentle Circumcision (quite a misleading name!) lists costs ranging from $250 to $450 for infants under 12 months old, to $1,600 for those over 18 years of age.[20]

As mentioned earlier, adult circumcisions are more costly because they often involve general anesthesia, the use of which is avoided in infants, meaning that infant circumcisions always involve inadequate pain relief, with the subsequent lower cost coming at the expense of humane treatment.

Many places provide coverage for circumcision in their social health care programs, meaning taxpayers often foot the bill for unnecessary circumcisions.[21] Some insurance providers also cover circumcision, even when it isn't medically necessary (which is most of the time), meaning that their customers ultimately pay higher premiums to cover the cost.

Circumcision service providers also routinely downplay the risks and exaggerate the benefits to get customers through their doors. The Queensland Circumcision Service in Australia is but one example. On its website it says, "We promise that you will go home with a SMILE on your face after your circumcision procedure!" which it also describes being "pain free"[22] (at least until the anesthetic wears off).

For all the trumped-up claims of medical benefits, private clinics like these show that circumcision is almost always a cosmetic procedure that in addition to costing men their foreskin also costs an arm and a leg.[23] But the money to be made from circumcision doesn't end with the bill for the surgery. Indeed, the integrity of the medical profession isn't the only thing for sale – the foreskins are too.

Foreskin facials

Foreskins contain cells called fibroblasts, and harvested foreskins can be stored in culture media (designed to support the growth of cells or microorganisms) for 24 days and still produce viable, functioning fibroblasts.[24] It is these cells that make foreskins a valuable commodity. Biotech companies sell vials containing half a million foreskin-derived fibroblasts for anything from a few to several hundred dollars.[25]

The reason fibroblasts are valuable is because they produce the skin-firming protein collagen, as well as another protein called elastin, which helps the skin keep its shape despite mechanical forces like pulling or stretching. Fibroblasts also produce hyaluronic acid, which helps trap moisture in the skin, and an enzyme which breaks down proteins in scar tissue. Add all that up and you've got the holy grail of skin treatments. One such popular skin treatment containing fibroblasts derived from infant foreskins, according to one retailer, contains about 20 million fibroblasts per milliliter and costs roughly $1,000 (USD),[26] which sounds like a bargain when you consider biotech companies are selling a vial of only half a million cells for several hundred dollars.

Fibroblasts aren't just used in cosmetics. They are also used as feeder cells to support the growth of human embryonic stem cells,[27] to produce interferon,[28] which is used to treat various cancers and viral infections, and in products that assist wound healing. For example, Dermagraft® is a skin substitute used to treat diabetic ulcers that contains foreskin-derived fibroblasts.[29] All that might make it sound like foreskin fibroblasts are incredibly useful, and they are, but fibroblasts can be derived from other tissues, not just foreskin. The main reason foreskin tissue is such a common source of fibroblasts is that foreskins are in such large supply due to circumcision.

So just how much is a foreskin worth? Canadian doctor Paul Tinari – who in 2006 successfully sued the British Columbian Ministry of Health to cover most of the cost of his foreskin restoration surgery (he was forcibly circumcised by school doctors at the age of 8) – estimates that between the surgery and resale value of a foreskin, each foreskin is worth $100,000.[30] That's quite a large number, and its accuracy is certainly debatable. I suspect he arrived at such a large figure because fibroblasts from a single foreskin can be used to create long-lived cell lines that continue to reap profits. Indeed, through cell proliferation, a single foreskin can produce 250,000 square feet (or a bit over four U.S. football fields) of Dermagraft® tissue.[31]

While it is difficult to determine exactly how much money is being made from the sale of foreskin and foreskin-derived products, what is certain is that neither the parents of circumcised boys, nor the boys themselves, see a cut of the profits.

Everyone's a critic

Imagine if people acted the same way about art as they do about genital cutting. I happen to love impressionist artwork. I find it superior to any other form of art. So, I am going to nail an impressionist piece to your living room wall. You cannot ever remove it or move house. On second thought, instead I'm going to print you a t-shirt with the same impressionist piece on it. You must wear this t-shirt for the rest of your life. You can never take it off. Wait, no, I think it is best we have this impressionist piece tattooed on your body. It is only right that my aesthetic preference be permanently marked on your flesh. This is my gift to you. It must always be with you, whether you like it or not. If none of this sounds appealing, you now have some idea how many people feel when they discover their parents decided what the most intimate part of their body would look (and indeed feel) like for the rest of their lives.

Those who have had their genitals cut may learn to love it, but most merely tolerate or do their best to ignore it. Those who are positively happy with their cut genitals tend to be those who made their own decision to have them surgically altered. But a word of warning to anyone who may be considering cosmetic genital surgery to appease others: change yourself for someone else and you'll soon learn that everyone's a critic. Just as it is impossible to grow parts of your genitals back, it is impossible to please everyone, and those you change yourself for are likely to demand even more.

...

All matters of appearance are viewed with a degree of subjectivity, which is precisely why cosmetic operations in general, and of the genitals in particular, should be a decision left to the individual whose body is going under the knife. Just as thinking a certain form of art looks better does not confer upon one a right to force it on others, so too thinking a particular surgical alteration of the genitals is more aesthetically pleasing does not give one a right to force it on others. Whether or not genital cutting spoils the appearance of a person, and is thus considered disfiguring, is a matter for the individual to decide. Infants and children should be allowed to grow up and decide for themselves whether they think cutting their genitals will improve the aesthetic down there.

6

Copy cuts

I suspect readers would be horrified by the notion of breaking the bones in a young girl's feet and forcing her to wear restrictive shoes day and night, ensuring that as her feet grew, they became so deformed they resembled hooves. How could anyone even think of doing such a thing, you might well be wondering. And yet as many readers will know, the hideous practice I have just described, known as footbinding, was a common practice in China for over a thousand years. Mothers whose feet were bound continued the practice by binding the feet of their daughters in a cycle of abuse that lasted many generations, until it finally fell out of favor in the early twentieth century. Only a handful of elderly women survive with their feet bound today, but that there are living survivors of this horrific practice at all stands as a reminder of how recently it came to an end.

Footbinding on its own is bad enough, but the reason countless women were made to suffer through the lifelong disability that came with having their feet crushed and deformed only makes the suffering they endured more tragic. Footbinding was practiced because many believed it made women more sexually appealing. According to Beverley Jackson, the author of *Splendid Slippers: A Thousand Years of An Erotic Tradition*, the weight constantly being carried by a foot-bound woman's heels forced her to walk with a particular posture and gait that meant the muscles in her legs, hips and vagina tightened, the result being that some Chinese men "claimed making love to a woman with bound feet was like making love to a virgin every time."[1]

If the notion of inflicting a permanent body modification on a child so they are one day able to meet the sexual desires of adults sounds familiar, it should, because that is precisely the reason given for cutting the genitals of millions of children today. There are many who say the genital cutting of girls is more pleasing to men and improves their marital eligibility, and there are also many who say circumcised penises are more attractive to women (and indeed also to men). Often it is the parents who advance such sexually charged arguments when justifying the cutting of their children's genitals.[2] I cannot profess to know why it is so important to some parents that their son have as similar a penis as possible to the one they have,[3] or prefer to have sex with, but perhaps that is a question they should be asking themselves.

A study of 145 women from Iowa in the US sought to "determine if women, particularly mothers who recently made a decision about circumcision of their newborn sons, do indeed prefer circumcised sexual partners, and if so, for what reasons."[4] Responding to the question, "If you could choose anyone for your ideal male sex partner, which circumcision type would you prefer he have for the following activities?" 71% preferred sex with circumcised penises, 76% preferred the look of them, 75% preferred giving circumcised penises "manual stimulation" and 83% preferred giving circumcised penises fellatio.[5] Also interesting is that when asked, "Why do you prefer one penis type over another for sex?" 92% said it is because it "stays cleaner", 90% because it "looks sexier", and 77% said because it "seems more natural."[6] These women were conflating "natural" with what they perceive as "normal". This survey was conducted in 1988, and attitudes in Iowa may have changed since then, but as intact men are often rudely reminded, there remain women in various parts of the world who have a sexual preference for circumcised penises, and who consider this on some level when deciding to circumcise their sons. I think it incredibly presumptuous of mothers who think circumcised penises look better to assume all other women think the same, or that their sons will even be attracted to women, much less care what they think about their having a foreskin.

I'm sure parents aren't actually visualizing their child's future sex life in any graphic detail, so much as they are thinking about their own sex lives and projecting them onto their children, in a sort of "what was good (or good enough) for me will be good for my child" line of thinking; a line of thinking that could also be taken the other way: "What was bad for me will be bad for my child." This perhaps explains why some intact fathers who were shamed for their foreskin by their peers and sexual partners circumcise their sons, to spare them the shaming they endured; or why some mothers, who have been the ones doing such shaming, circumcise their sons so other women won't treat them the same way they treated their own intact male partners. All this is ironic, because it perpetuates the very cause of the bullying some parents are concerned about, ensuring many more children will continue to suffer from it.

One of the lowlier aspects of human nature is the tendency to shame those who are different simply for being different. And as it happens, there are populations in which most men are circumcised, and in which those kept intact appear to be the ones who are different. But the shaming of intact men goes beyond their being different, because the very existence of intact men can be taken, and indeed is taken by many, as an affront to the normality of circumcision. And if circumcision isn't normal, then it is the circumcised men who are different (and by their own logic worthy of shame). Note, however, that the shaming does not go both ways, for there is not widespread shaming of men with circumcised penises in majority intact populations. This is not surprising. After all, intact men have nothing to prove, and few would stoop so low as to shame a victim of genital mutilation.

Compare this to majority circumcised populations such as the US, in which shaming of intact penises permeates popular culture, and regularly makes its way into popular TV shows. Take *Sex and the City*, for example, a show premised on sexual liberation that somehow still managed to be sexually repressive on several occasions. In season 2, episode 9, an episode crudely titled "Old Dogs, New Dicks", the prudish character Charlotte is so repulsed by her new lover's foreskin that she refers to it as the "Shar-Pei" (a breed of dog known for its distinctive deep wrinkles). Her lover confesses he has had the same bad reaction from his previous partners and decides to get circumcised. When Charlotte sees his newly circumcised penis she declares, "It's perfect!" (Apparently nothing says perfection like scar tissue.) Toward the end of the episode, now feeling sexually liberated for the first time in his life, Charlotte's lover leaves her to go and play the field. This sorry affair is not confined to television. It plays itself out again daily in the lives of men and women the world over; men and women who are shamed by others for not conforming to their expectations of what constitutes "normal".

The pressure to conform of course goes beyond the appearance of our genitals – it intrudes on every aspect of our lives. While in many cases people acquiescing to society's standards can be a good thing – for example, the social pressure on people to bathe regularly so they don't expose others to unpleasant odors – we must not tolerate forcing things on others that cause them harm. Consent matters. It is why putting a lit cigarette in a child's mouth and telling them to smoke is child abuse, but an adult choosing to smoke cigarettes in full knowledge of the harm they are causing themselves is acceptable. The fundamental problem with non-consensual genital cutting is not that it's harmful, but rather that it's forced on individuals without their informed consent.

Problems with conformist arguments

The notion that because most people in some populations have had their genitals cut, the minority who haven't should also have their genitals cut, is a conformist argument. Conformist arguments often contain an appeal to tradition, because if a practice is common in a community, it's often because people have been doing it for some time. And the mere fact a practice has been performed for a long time is used as an excuse for its continuation. Indeed, proponents of circumcision love reminding us that circumcision has been performed for thousands of years, but so what? The foreskin evolved millions of years ago, so it has been around a lot longer than the several thousand years some have been cutting it off. Appeals to tradition are fallacious, because the fact something has been done for a long time does not guarantee that it's a good practice. Footbinding was around for a long time, and it was bloody horrible.

The conformist argument does not need to rely on a fallacious appeal to tradition. For many it is simply enough that circumcision is commonplace in the present to warrant its practice. This is an appeal to popularity, and it's also fallacious, because the mere fact a practice is popular doesn't guarantee it's a good practice. In the sixteenth century the French burned cats alive to the delight of crowds of spectators who "shrieked with laughter as the animals, howling with pain, were signed, roasted, and finally carbonized."[7] Today it is difficult to find anyone who would publicly condone such barbarism, but the French would probably still be burning cats alive today if they thought just because it was a popular practice in the sixteenth century that it should continue to enjoy popularity.

Like father like son

It is not unusual to hear fathers say things like, "I want my son to look like me", when defending their decision to circumcise their sons. And if you think the parental decision to circumcise sons so they match a male relative is uncommon, think again. Studies have found it to be one of the most common factors, if not the most common factor, influencing the parental decision to circumcise.[8] To circumcise a boy so his genitals match those of another male relative is the most vacuous and narcissistic of all the arguments in favor of circumcision, and curiously a majority see nothing wrong with it. But imagine if parents said, "I want my child to look like me" before giving their baby a tattoo. No one would think that a normal, sane thing to do. And yet just like circumcision, tattooing is a painful procedure, the consequences of which are permanent (barring expensive and painful laser surgery).

What's interesting is that violating another's bodily autonomy is generally considered socially unacceptable even when the consequences aren't permanent. Consider that if I were to cut someone's hair in a style of my choosing without their consent (say I were to do so while they slept), because in my view this particular hairstyle was better than what they already had, or because I wanted our hairstyles to match, I would rightly be regarded as domineering if not totally insane. I fail to see how cutting the genitals of another without their consent is any different, except that unlike hair, genitals do not grow back. To be clear, I am *not* suggesting that parents have no right to cut their children's hair; a right they clearly have even when children throw a tantrum and don't want a haircut. What I am suggesting is that we afford more moral consideration and significance to adults cutting each other's hair than we do to adults cutting children's genitals, and that this is inversely proportional to the moral weight and harm each carries. If I cut another adult's hair without their consent, I could potentially find myself in court, even though their hair will grow back, and I have caused them no harm beyond perhaps a little social embarrassment. But if I were to have a son and cut off his foreskin, I would likely face no legal consequences, despite the fact his foreskin will never grow back, and I would have caused him physical harm.

Given the permanent nature of circumcision, and the potential for the procedure to go disastrously wrong (as detailed in Chapter 4), you might expect circumcision to be a heavily regulated practice, but such an expectation is far from reality. Indeed, in the US anyone can legally perform ritual male circumcision.[9] By contrast, hygienic practices as relatively trivial as hair or nail cutting are heavily regulated.[10]

Circumcised prospective fathers who plan to circumcise their sons so they match should ask themselves if it *really* is that important that their son have a similar-looking penis. They should imagine what they would do if their son's circumcision was botched (say the procedure resulted in an amputated or buried penis). Would it still be as important to the father that they match? Would he be eagerly awaiting surgery to amputate or bury his penis so that he matches his son? Or would this trivial and bizarre concern that their penises match like an ugly pair of earrings immediately vanish, and be replaced by feelings of anger toward, and a lawsuit against, their son's doctor? The latter is of course what happens in such cases, because fundamentally circumcised men don't really want their sons' penises to match their own, what they want is to act like circumcision is a "normal" thing for parents to force on their children, and in so doing justify what was done to them. So, while anger against doctors who botch circumcisions is warranted (and one might add also warranted for those that perform unnecessary circumcisions whether botched or not), let's not scapegoat the doctors. Any parent who consents to their son having a medically unnecessary circumcision, despite knowing the risks and harms of the procedure, is also responsible. Accepting that responsibility is a hard thing to do, but it is the right thing to do.

Teasing in the locker room

Many parents desire for their sons to fit in with their peers, and express concern they will be teased in the locker room if they aren't circumcised like the other boys. According to a study of male students at the University of Iowa, this concern appears to be not entirely unfounded.[11] The students answered a questionnaire about their middle and high school locker room experience, to determine whether they witnessed others being teased or were teased themselves about the appearance of their penis.[12] As rates of circumcision in the Midwest are higher than anywhere else in the United States, it is not surprising that 87% of respondents were circumcised. If there were anywhere you'd expect to see intact men teased for having a foreskin this would be the place.[13] Interestingly, even though most men were circumcised, most teasing related to penis size, with 75% of respondents having been teased, and 83% having witnessed someone else being teased, about the size of their member. Only 24% of teasing witnessed in the locker room related to having a foreskin, and you'd expect this number to be even lower in places where circumcision is less common.

All this paints a picture of a truly bizarre situation, in which some parents cut their sons' genitals to prevent them being teased for not being cut, which rarely happens and wouldn't happen at all if it weren't for so many other parents cutting their sons in the first place; and all this despite the fact they will be teased about their genitals anyway, and much more frequently as far as size is concerned. What's more, despite the occasional teasing, the vast majority of intact men reported that they liked their penis the way it is and wouldn't change it, a fact that supports their parents' decision not to circumcise them.

Counting the cutting

If the fact intact men are rarely teased for having a foreskin still isn't enough to convince some parents that they shouldn't circumcise their sons, then such parents should remember the conformist argument only makes sense in places circumcision is widespread to begin with.

On the one hand, in countries with an already high circumcision rate, conformist thinking works in favor of circumcising boys. On the other hand, in countries with a low circumcision rate, it works in favor of leaving boys part of the intact majority. But talk of the circumcision "rate" can be confusing, because it could refer either to prevalence (the total number of boys and men who are circumcised in a population), or incidence (the number of newly circumcised boys and men each year).

The circumcision rate is often very different when one is talking in terms of prevalence or incidence. Parents in a country like Australia, for example, should be aware that although the circumcision rate in terms of prevalence is still quite high, the circumcision rate in terms of incidence is relatively low. This means that even though most men might still be circumcised, most in their son's peer group will not be, and within a couple of generations the prevalence of circumcision will lower to resemble the incidence, assuming no change in current trends. This line of reasoning may cause parents in Australia to leave their sons intact, yet at the same time cause parents in the US to circumcise their sons, because the circumcision rate in terms of incidence is still a majority there (albeit a slim one due to the decline in newborn circumcisions there over the past decade). I think the fact that the argument from conformity can be used to support or oppose circumcision shows how vacuous it is.

As a matter of principle, children should be allowed to grow up and decide whether they conform in the way their parents do, or not. In practice, however, there will always be some parents who circumcise their sons for conformist reasons. If you count yourself among them, remember that most men worldwide are not circumcised,[14] and consider that the incidence and prevalence of circumcision varies greatly according to location. In 2010 the Royal Australasian College of Physicians estimated that 10–20% of Australian newborn boys were circumcised.[15] Meanwhile a survey conducted in Canada estimated that in 2006–2007, the circumcision of newborns was 31.9%.[16] In both Australia and Canada the circumcision rate varied greatly (and still does) from one state or territory to another. In Australia, data from 2010 showed that Tasmania had the lowest newborn circumcision rate at 1.5%, and New South Wales had the highest at 17.3%.[17] In Canada, data from 2006 to 2007 showed Nova Scotia had the lowest newborn circumcision rate at 6.8%, and Alberta had the highest at 44.3%.[18] Such marked regional variation means talk of national circumcision rates is misleading parents.

How do we go about explaining the relatively large differences in circumcision rates between regions of the same country? The reduction of newborn circumcisions in some places reflects, in part, an increasing public awareness that the procedure is unnecessary and harmful. But there is evidence to suggest that in the US, at least, the decrease in circumcision rates to date has been due to a passive demographic shift rather than an active cultural one against the practice. The Centers for Disease Control and Prevention attributed the decline of newborn circumcisions in the western United States from 62% in 1980 to 37% in 1999 to the increased birth rate of the Hispanic population, who are less likely to circumcise. Rates in the Northeast for the same time period remained roughly the same with a small decline from 67 to 66%, and increased in the South from 56 to 64%, and the Midwest from 76 to 81%.[19] We also know from a study conducted in 2009 that the incidence of circumcision in rural areas for that year was 66.9%, much higher than the 41.2% in urban areas.[20] This shows that while the majority of newborns in the US are currently circumcised, the higher circumcision rates in rural areas are pushing up the national average, with a majority of newborns in cities already kept intact.

A cut above the rest

The high national circumcision rate in the US is almost unique among secular developed countries. I say "almost unique" because there is one other developed country with a high male circumcision rate not due to the presence of a large Muslim or Jewish population: South Korea. Circumcision was virtually non-existent in South Korea until the involvement of the US in the Korean War and the immense cultural influence that followed. Koreans came to view circumcision as a mark of an advanced modern culture and were quick to adopt the practice.

A study of 1,674 South Korean men conducted in 2001 reported four interesting findings: 1) that 78% of those surveyed were circumcised, with a further 11.5% of intact men wishing to become circumcised; 2) in stark contrast to the US, only 1% of circumcisions were performed on males within a year of birth, with most being performed around the age of puberty; 3) that despite their age, and 82.8% of men who responded saying the decision of the child ought to be the most important, the decision to circumcise was still made by the parents in 67.4% of cases; and 4) that 71.1% of the men surveyed thought circumcision improved penile hygiene, but more than half reported no knowledge regarding a range of proposed medical benefits.[21]

The results of another study of 3,296 South Korean men conducted from 2009 to 2011 indicated the prevalence of circumcision had been in sharp decline over the preceding decade when compared to previous results from a 2002 study, dropping from 95.2 to 74.4% in boys aged 17–19, and from 88.4 to 56.4% in those aged 14–16.[22] The researchers noted that circumcision was originally adopted in South Korea in spite of tradition and in the absence of any clear medical benefits. They attributed its decline to education and greater access to information about the history of circumcision in the country. This stands in contrast to the US, where demographic shifts appear to have been the main driver of change. South Korea remains a case in point about why it is unwise to adopt a practice – especially one that involves removing a part of your anatomy – for the purpose of "keeping up with the Joneses", or in this case, the Johnsons, rather than due consideration of the evidence.

Another country in which circumcision used to be popular, but has since fallen out of favor, is the United Kingdom. There are various reasons put forward for how male circumcision became common in the UK. It is often said that the British royal family has a tradition of circumcision dating back to Queen Victoria, who it is asserted believed herself to be a descendant of King David (the David who slew Goliath). Indeed, for this reason there was much media speculation surrounding the fate of Prince William's son's foreskin shortly after his birth in 2013; speculation that is misinformed, because it is a myth that the royal family traditionally circumcises its male members' members.

Princes William and Harry are most likely intact, although their father King Charles is most likely circumcised.[23] It would seem King Charles and other British Royals before him were circumcised because circumcision was "a common practice among the British middle and wealthy classes from the 1890s to the 1940s, widely recommended as a sensible hygienic precaution, and the monarchy was following middle class fashion and the prevailing medical wisdom."[24] The myth of a circumcision tradition dating back to Queen Victoria entertaining fantasies of a Davidic lineage is an urban legend popularized by the late Edgar Schoen, an American physician and long-time proponent of male circumcision.[25] How much this myth has contributed to those who've heard it choosing to circumcise their sons remains unclear, but what is clear is that central to the popularity of genital cutting (especially male circumcision), is that it is seen to serve as a physical mark of social distinction.

A common thread in both religious and medical discourse promoting genital cutting is the same today as it has been for centuries: purity. As Mary Douglas expounded upon in her book, *Purity and Danger: An Analysis of Concepts of Pollution and Taboo*, cleanliness and uncleanliness are just another measure of a person's place in the social hierarchy.[26] As the medical historian David Gollaher once put it, "Class distinction ... assumed growing importance around the turn of the [twentieth] century ... Outside Judaism, circumcision was exclusively the province of doctors and patients with enough money to pay for an elective procedure."[27] The result of this combination of connotations of purity and the backing of the medical profession was that, to quote Gollaher again, medical circumcision "assumed its own place in the fin-de-siècle search for rank and social order ... It signified precisely that aversion to dirt – and not just dirt, but vulgarity, nasty habits, and diseases – which symbolically set one on a higher plane."[28]

...

"Like mother like daughter" is no excuse for footbinding or female genital mutilation, and "like father like son" is no excuse for circumcision. It is not okay to permanently alter another person's body without their consent to suit the preferences or desires of others. People have no more a right to mutilate the genitals of children now than they had to mutilate the feet of young girls, which to be clear, is no right at all. Even if genital cutting conveys social benefits, it is neither the role of parents nor medical professionals to act as judge, jury, and excisioner.

7

On religious freedom, rights, and the law

My old fencing master, Cornel Vena, who defected from communist Romania at the 1956 Melbourne Olympics to live as a free man in Australia, once told me he came to realize there's no freedom in life, only in death. I disagreed, because the dead cannot experience freedom, unless one thinks of "freedom" as an inability to experience anything, but I understood the point he was making. In communist Romania his freedom was limited because those with power had taken it from him and the rest of the Romanian working class, whereas in a capitalist country like Australia, he found he was only as free as he could afford to be. He had traded being a slave to people for being a slave to the dollar. Although this is far from ideal, most people accept this as a pretty good trade-off so long as they can afford to live comfortably.

While attempts to erode our fundamental freedoms remain, they are, by and large, protected in free societies, which is why we refer to those societies as such. However, even in free societies our freedoms are not without limits. For example, we accept that we're not free to drive on whatever side of the road we want to, or pilot aircraft with no prior training. We accept limits to our freedom to avoid threats to the health and safety of ourselves and others. It's curious then that so many turn a blind eye to the genital cutting of children, particularly when done for religious reasons, as if religion granted a chosen few a God-given right to harm others. Imagine if some people claimed a right to cut off their children's little fingers or toes, or to use the example of something seemingly less important, their earlobes. (Unlike the foreskin, earlobes actually are useless flaps of skin.) Imagine further that by some accident of history this teaching had been enshrined in scripture, and that some religious people were today claiming a right to cut off their children's earlobes. Most people would not tolerate this, so why do so many make an exception when it comes to cutting off parts of genitals, which unlike earlobes have important functions? And why do so many who would never make this exception for girls make it for boys?

Many parents who circumcise their sons for religious reasons also claim it's supported by medical benefits, suggesting that tacitly they recognize religious grounds alone cannot justify their actions. Of course, there are also many who claim the right to cut their children's genitals even in the absence of medical benefits, or even in the knowledge it is harmful, and who argue that any attempt to stop them from doing so is a violation of their religious freedom. After all, freedom of religion is a right protected under international human rights law, guaranteed by the First Amendment of the Constitution of the United States of America, and that is provided for in one way or another in many other countries. There's no doubt that freedom of religion is important. Our modern-day secular liberal democracies couldn't function without it. However, like freedom in general, religious freedom has its limits. The only question is where to draw the line, and it is reasonable to draw that line at harming others.

In 2012, a regional court in Cologne, Germany, ruled that non-therapeutic male circumcision – even when properly performed by a doctor – is an illegal procedure that causes bodily harm.[1] The case related to the circumcision of a four-year-old boy, who was cut by a doctor not for any medical reason, but because his Muslim parents decided he should be. The court also ruled that parental consent was insufficient, because parental rights do not include the right to consent to a procedure that isn't in the child's best interests, and that circumcision was not in the child's best interests, not "even for the purposes of avoiding a possible exclusion from their religious community and the parental right of education."[2] Finally, the court ruled that the permanent and irreparable change to the child's body "runs contrary to the interests of the child in deciding his religious affiliation independently later in life."[3] This ruling generated heated protests from Jews and Muslims, and the Merkel government rushed to pass a new law clarifying that: 1) medically unnecessary male circumcision of boys too young to consent is legal when performed by a doctor with parental consent; 2) parents forcing their children to undergo religious male circumcision is covered by their parental rights; and 3) religious circumcisions can be performed by trained religious practitioners who are not doctors.[4]

So ingrained is circumcision in Judaism, that any opposition to it is almost certain to see one charged with being antisemitic. German politicians are understandably especially sensitive to this,[5] which is why when it came to the debate over male circumcision and the Cologne ruling, they didn't walk on eggshells so much as hover over them. There is, however, a difference between a hatred of the Jewish people, which is clearly antisemitic, and opposition to the practice of circumcision, which is not a sufficient condition of antisemitism; if it were then the many Jewish people who oppose circumcision would absurdly also have to be considered antisemitic.

Most people who reject male circumcision are not antisemitic, which is why they reject not just Jewish circumcision, but any form of genital cutting performed on minors in the absence of their own informed consent or medical necessity. This was the position of the Association of Pediatricians in Germany, which outlined in its submission on Germany's draft ritual circumcision bill, that "there is no reason from a medical point of view to remove an intact foreskin from underage boys or boys unable to give consent."[6] Despite the protestations of religious lobby groups and the capitulation of the German government, the ruling of the court in Cologne remains in line with international human rights law.

Non-consensual, medically unnecessary genital cutting violates human rights

Human rights are international legal norms that transcend social, cultural, national and religious differences.[7] According to Article 5 of the Vienna Declaration and Programme of Action, adopted at the World Conference on Human Rights in Vienna in 1993, "all human rights are universal, indivisible and interdependent and interrelated, [and they must be treated equally] on the same footing, and with the same emphasis."[8] These rights are set out in a number of legally binding treaties, including the International Covenant on Civil and Political Rights, the International Covenant on Economic, Social and Cultural Rights, the European Convention on Human Rights, the Convention against Torture, and the Convention on the Rights of the Child.[9]

It is well established that female genital mutilation violates human rights.[10] There is, however, an emerging legal view that non-consensual, medically unnecessary male circumcision also violates human rights, and that religious freedom isn't a valid justification for this violation.[11] There are, of course, some who disagree. They cite the right of parents not just to freedom of religion, but to ensure their children's education is consistent with their religious and moral convictions.[12] All well and good, except as human rights law makes clear, this right may be limited to protect children's human rights and fundamental freedoms,[13] and non-consensual, medically unnecessary genital cutting is in breach of multiple human rights. It violates the right to freedom from all forms of violence,[14] the right to security of person,[15] the right to freedom from torture or cruel, inhuman, or degrading treatment or punishment,[16] the right to the highest attainable standard of health,[17] and when done for religious reasons to a child too young to consent, it violates the child's right to freedom of thought, conscience and religion.[18]

The right to freedom from all forms of violence includes freedom from "all forms of physical or mental violence, injury or abuse, neglect or negligent treatment, [and] maltreatment or exploitation, including sexual abuse."[19] In defining such harmful practices, we "must in no way erode the child's absolute right to human dignity and physical and psychological integrity by describing some forms of violence as legally and/or socially acceptable."[20] Harmful practices, including non-consensual, medically unnecessary genital cutting, are a violation of the right to freedom from all forms of violence.

The right to security of person exists to safeguard personal integrity and protect individuals against intentional infliction of bodily or mental injury.[21] Since genital cutting always results in some degree of bodily harm, and often results in mental harm, it is clearly in violation of the right to security of person. Parents have a great deal of freedom when it comes to raising their children in accordance with their own cultural and religious beliefs. However, the best interests of the child must be their primary concern,[22] and non-consensual, medically unnecessary genital cutting is not in any child's best interests, because it is harmful and prejudicial to their bodily integrity and autonomy.

The Committee on the Rights of the Child makes it clear that the right to freedom from torture or cruel, inhuman, or degrading treatment or punishment includes freedom from "all forms of physical or mental violence [and] violence in the guise of treatment."[23] Acts that are not within the scope of torture may be considered cruel, inhuman, or degrading treatment or punishment (hereafter collectively "ill treatment"). The distinction between torture and ill treatment is determined not by the intensity of the pain or suffering inflicted, but by the intent of the act and the powerlessness of the victim.[24] Female genital mutilation is roundly accepted as a form of torture and ill treatment under human rights law.[25] In 2013 and 2016, the Special Rapporteur on Torture stated that non-consensual, medically unnecessary body modifications of intersex people – who have innate variations in sex characteristics that mean they are not typically male or female – are likewise a form of torture and ill treatment, and called for them to be outlawed.[26] I believe that non-consensual, medically unnecessary male genital cutting also violates the right of the child to freedom from torture and ill treatment. Importantly, any actual or perceived *medical benefits* of male circumcision or medical interventions on intersex children and young people cannot justify such practices, because the medicalization of harmful practices does not absolve the violation of human rights.[27] Indeed, the only time such practices should be permitted without an individual's informed consent is when their informed consent cannot be obtained and the medical intervention being performed is *medically necessary*.

The right to the highest attainable standard of health includes sexual and reproductive health, as well as the right to bodily autonomy.[28] The Convention of the Rights of the Child specifies that ratifying states must "take all effective and appropriate measures with a view to abolishing traditional practices prejudicial to the health of children."[29] Even if male circumcision does convey some minor health benefits, there is no denying it is also prejudicial to health in a number of ways, and that it carries the risk of complications; nor is there any denying that the overwhelming view of the international medical community is that these benefits do not outweigh the risks. Countries have an obligation to ensure the healthy development of children and to reduce infant mortality,[30] and medically unnecessary genital cutting poses avoidable risks to the healthy development and lives of children. Indeed, in the US it accounts for 1.3% of all infant male deaths.[31] In their efforts to progressively realize the right to health, countries must commit resources and engage in international cooperation.[32] However, global initiatives that promote male circumcision for its claimed population health benefits, in particular the claim it reduces female-to-male HIV transmission, do so despite a lack of conclusive evidence or medical consensus (see Chapter 3), and at the expense of upholding human rights.[33]

The right to freedom of thought, conscience, and religion "can never be legitimately invoked to justify the infliction of grave and often traumatic violations of a person's physical and psychological integrity."[34] And this right applies as much to children as it does to their parents or guardians. To be clear, although the Convention on the Rights of the Child deals explicitly with the rights of children, the rights outlined in other treaties also apply to children as much as they do to adults. This is important to recognize, because at the heart of this argument is the unspoken false assumption that the right to freedom of religion only applies to adults, and more specifically to parents but not their children. However, since children are also human beings, they also have rights, and they enjoy these rights independently from their parents. In other words, children are individual bearers of rights, because children are people, not the property of their parents.[35]

Unless religious freedom applies to everyone there is no freedom of religion, only the privileging of some religious people and their beliefs over others. That's why human rights law makes it clear that the right to freedom of religion (like all other human rights) applies to everyone, and why freedom of religion ought to be conveyed to every single individual, young or old. The religious genital cutting of children too young to consent is a breach of their right to freedom of religion because it denies them the opportunity to decide for themselves if they wish to take part in a religious ritual that involves the permanent removal of part of their body. Children that are too young to understand theological concepts ought to be allowed to grow up and, when they're old enough, choose religious beliefs or practices, or the lack thereof, for themselves.[36] It is not okay to force a religious practice on someone at knifepoint.

On the illegality of genital cutting

We've seen that non-consensual, medically unnecessary genital cutting violates human rights, but those who perform it may also be breaking the law. Many countries have introduced laws banning female genital mutilation. Unfortunately, at the time of this writing, not a single country has passed laws that explicitly prohibit non-consensual, medically unnecessary male genital cutting, and only Malta has banned non-consensual, medically unnecessary modifications of intersex minors' bodies.[37] There is a view in some jurisdictions, however, that non-consensual, medically unnecessary male circumcision and intersex body modifications are already illegal under common law, and increasingly legal bodies and scholars are calling for these practices to be made illegal, or for the law to be clarified to make it clear that they already are.

In Australia, the Queensland Law Reform Commission concluded in a 1993 report that non-therapeutic circumcision without the consent of the individual being circumcised is unlawful under common law, and that it could be regarded as a criminal act under specific laws relating to assault and injury.[38] In 2012, the Tasmania Law Reform Institute recommended a legal prohibition on non-therapeutic male circumcision, with limited, highly regulated exemptions for religious and cultural observance.[39]

In 2013, the Council of Europe passed a resolution, which is not legally binding, that declared male circumcision performed for religious reasons, along with female genital mutilation and early childhood medical interventions on intersex children, to be a "a violation of the physical integrity of children."[40] In the same year, the Nordic Association of Children's Ombudsmen and pediatric experts issued a statement calling all involved parties to "work towards a situation where circumcision without medical indication may only be carried out if a boy, who has reached the age and maturity required in order to understand the necessary medical information, chooses to consent to the procedure."[41]

A few court rulings in European countries are also of interest. In addition to the Cologne ruling in 2012, German courts have ruled in 2007 and 2013, respectively, that circumcision is an unlawful personal injury,[42] and that parental consent is not valid if the possible psychological damage circumcision might cause the child is not considered.[43] In 2015, in a case concerning female genital cutting, a UK judge in the Royal Court of Justice stated that if, as was their view, type IV female genital mutilation causes significant harm, then the same must also be said of male circumcision.[44] In 2016, a UK judge in the High Court of Justice refused to permit the circumcision of two boys of Muslim parents, noting that circumcision carries risks, that nothing in Islam mandates circumcision before an age where the boys could consent to be circumcised themselves, and that while remaining intact the boys could fully participate in the Muslim community and culture.[45]

In South Africa, the law prohibits circumcision of males under the age of 16 except when performed for religious purposes, or for medical reasons on the recommendation of a medical practitioner.[46] Notably, "medical reasons" is not limited to medical *necessity*, making this legislation symbolic and ineffectual, since an argument for medical benefits, however slim, can always be made.

In the US, Congress banned non-therapeutic female genital cutting in 1996, and stated in its findings that it "infringes upon the guarantees of rights secured by Federal and State law, both statutory and constitutional."[47] In other words, female genital cutting was already unlawful under particular state and federal laws, which means the genital cutting of boys is also already unlawful under those laws.[48] Congress also stated in its findings that "the practice of female genital mutilation is carried out by certain cultural and religious groups within the United States," which notably wasn't viewed as a valid reason to have religious exemptions to the ban. Well-intentioned though legislators are, state and federal laws against female genital mutilation discriminate on the basis of sex, and violate the Equal Protection Clause of state and federal constitutions, as well as international law.[49] Indeed, in late 2018 a federal judge ruled the 1996 law prohibiting female genital mutilation was an unconstitutional form of sex-based discrimination, and argued that it was never not a crime to cut the healthy genitals of a non-consenting person, because that is a form of criminal assault already illegal in all fifty states in the US.[50]

Although circumcision of male minors is not commonly thought of as being child abuse, it certainly appears to fit the usual legal definition of it. Child abuse is commonly defined as the intentional use of force to injure a child, and is universally proscribed by state law.[51] To take one state as an example, in California the cutting of female genitals, however slight, is considered felony child abuse;[52] and medically unnecessary male circumcision also appears to meet the legal definition of child abuse, as well as of assault, battery, sexual abuse and sexual assault, leaving those who perform it potentially open to criminal prosecution.[53] However, circumcisers are to various degrees protected from the threat of prosecution in at least ten states by statutory and regulatory exemptions.[54] For example, Idaho,[55] Illinois[56] and Mississippi[57] all have statutes banning "ritual abuse" that exempt male circumcision, while Delaware,[58] Minnesota,[59] Montana[60] and Wisconsin[61] have exemptions permitting ritual circumcisers to practice medicine without a license.

Parental rights versus parental responsibilities

Clearly whatever rights parents have, these do not extend to breaking the law. If then, as appears to be the case in many jurisdictions, non-consensual, medically unnecessary male circumcision is already illegal, the question of the parental right to consent to it is moot. There is, however, an ongoing debate over the legalities of male circumcision in various jurisdictions throughout the world. Assuming one lives in a place non-consensual, medically unnecessary male circumcision is lawful, why shouldn't parents have a right to consent to it for their children? To answer this question, it is important to first understand that insofar as parental rights exist, they relate to parents raising their children without interference from the state. However, this requires parents to meet their parental responsibilities. When parents severely fail in their responsibility and breach their children's rights, parental rights are revoked, and children become wards of the state. This happens, for example, when parents beat their children. It does not happen, however, when they mutilate their genitals. If it did, half of all newborn boys in America would become wards of the state, which is not practical.

Aside from the impracticality of it, the reason we aren't calling social services every time a parent orders part of their son's genitals to be cut off is because we believe parents generally try to do what is in the best interests of their children, and that parents have a right to consent to medical procedures on their behalf. However, we've already seen medically unnecessary genital cutting is a harmful act not in any child's best interests, and while parents are often the people best placed to determine what is in the best interests of their children, this is not the case when it comes to genital cutting, particularly where parents have themselves been victims of it. As with most cycles of abuse, in an impulse to deny their own loss, the victims of genital cutting are often its strongest proponents.

Even if cut parents were well placed to make the circumcision decision, it still shouldn't be their decision to make. Parents often argue that circumcision is a "personal choice", but if they really believed this then they would respect the right of their child to make that personal choice for themselves when they are old enough to do so; they wouldn't argue, as many do, that the fact they know (or think they know) what's best gives them a right to overrule their child's autonomy. Imagine if doctors performed whatever procedures they wanted on patients without consent just because they know better and are better placed to be making such decisions. That would quite simply be unacceptable, not to mention illegal. Cutting the genitals of children too young to consent is likewise unacceptable and admits of only one exception – that an individual's informed consent cannot be obtained, and it is medically necessary.

The right of parents to make medical decisions, when they must for their children who are too young to take part in such decisions themselves, is not what is being questioned here. Parents undoubtedly have this right, but it is limited by their responsibility to protect their children's rights and do what is in their best interest. That's why parental rights are geared towards the protection of the rights of children. In other words, parents do not have *rights over* their children; they have *responsibilities to* their children, which include protecting their children's rights.

Some religious parents argue that stopping them from circumcising their children represents a breach of their right to freedom of religion, when at best it represents a limitation. This limitation is suitable and necessary to meet the legitimate objective of protecting children from the harms of genital cutting, and, on balance, prevents more harm than it causes. Permanent physical and, in many cases, psychological harm caused by genital cutting is averted. In exchange, one right is limited merely to the extent that some parents of some religious persuasions cannot mutilate their children's genitals. Most people in the developed world already accept that the right to freedom of religion cannot justify female genital mutilation, and their continuing to accept it as an excuse for male genital mutilation represents an indefensible double standard.

Rights can be widely accepted and recognized socially and legislated and recognized legally. Many people once claimed the right to own other human beings as property to be bought and sold, to subjugate women and exterminate people based on their ethnicity, religion, or sexuality. Some people still claim such rights even though human rights law explicitly forbids them from doing so, but such people are thankfully now in the minority, and ensuring they remain the minority requires eternal vigilance. Some people also still claim the right to mutilate the genitals of children. However, while there are many choices parents rightly get to make for their children, deciding how much of their body they get to keep should not be one of them.

Why circumcision should be unlawful

There are many who question the medical benefits and ethics of routine infant circumcision, or who question the legitimacy of ritual circumcision, yet who remain opposed to banning either practice. They reason that a ban will lead to an increase in unsafe backyard procedures. This was the very same reasoning behind the American Academy of Pediatrics' short-lived call in 2010 to legalize some forms of Type IV female genital mutilation in the US. It was a call briefly echoed in Australia, when the then secretary of The Royal Australian and New Zealand College of Obstetricians and Gynecologists (RANZCOG), Gino Pecoraro, jumped on the AAP bandwagon just as its wheels were falling off. In an article published on the 28th of March, Pecoraro is on record supporting the idea and saying, "No-one is condoning the practice. No-one is trying to legitimize the practice. They are trying to look at a way to minimize the harm."[62] The article was updated just three days later to say that the AAP had withdrawn its support for doctors to perform so-called "minor" forms of female genital cutting, and with that, Pecoraro and RANZCOG quietly withdrew their consideration and apparent provisional support for the idea as well.

Despite the abject refusal of the public to stomach the "harm minimization" argument for female genital mutilation, it's an argument that occasionally resurfaces in the media.[63] The danger is this argument appears on the surface like a rational one. It sounds reasonable to propose that although the genital mutilation of children is bad, it is better to have a "milder" version of the procedure performed by trained professionals (medical doctors) in controlled environments (hospitals) to minimize harm, until you consider what you are really being asked to condone. Imagine if someone told you that to stop family violence going on in the home, people should be brought to police stations, so that they can receive "milder" beatings by trained professionals (police officers) in controlled environments (police stations) to minimize harm. This is an utterly absurd and disgusting proposition, yet it is precisely the same logic put forward by those who want doctors to mutilate children to stem illegal backyard procedures. The reality is that if "no-one is condoning the practice" then no one should be willing to perform it; if "no-one is trying to legitimize the practice" then respectable medical organizations should not be putting their good names to it; and if you are a doctor trying to "minimize the harm", then you should do what your profession demands, and first, do no harm.

The fact is we cannot minimize harm by institutionalizing it. There is another fact we cannot ignore, too: prohibition doesn't work. It did not work for alcohol, and it is not working now in the failed war on other drugs. There is, however, a significant difference between prohibiting the consumption of a product by an individual who chooses to consume it and prohibiting the mutilation of the genitals of defenseless children who have no say in the matter.

How is it possible to live in a society in which no one thinks twice about parents mutilating the genitals of their children, or paying someone else to do so, but in which parents can also be imprisoned and have the custody of their children revoked for taking a knife to *any other part* of their body? In a more rational world, when parents solicit the services of a doctor to mutilate their children's genitals, the doctor would call social services and the police, not proceed to carry out the mutilation on their behalf for a fee. Sadly, many people, including some doctors, do not realize the harm they are causing, and therefore a ban, even though it is a moral imperative, won't work.

The fact a ban won't work, however, is not a valid reason for why there shouldn't be one. We have laws against all sorts of things and people break them all the time. As was once aptly noted by Paul Mason, former Commissioner for Children in Tasmania, and my predecessor as the founding chairperson of The Darbon Institute, we have laws against murder and people still commit murder, and yet no one would argue outlawing murder is pointless because it doesn't eliminate murder.[64] Laws like these serve as deterrents, imperfect to be sure, but deterrents, nonetheless. They also help promote a cultural shift against practices by establishing opposition to them as legal norms. Murder being illegal has clearly not eliminated murder, just as laws against female genital mutilation have not eliminated the butchering of female genitalia; and extending such laws to protect boys likewise won't end non-consensual, medically unnecessary male circumcision, but it is a good place to start.

While female genital mutilation is already a criminal offence in many places, many of those same jurisdictions will consider alternatives to criminalizing non-consensual, medically unnecessary male circumcision and intersex body modifications. This is problematic because, as we've seen, criminal laws against female genital mutilation can be on shaky legal ground for being a form of sex-based discrimination that breaches the right to non-discrimination. A consistent legal and regulatory approach to non-consensual, medically unnecessary and deferrable alterations of sex characteristics such as genital cutting, regardless of sex or gender, is needed. For several reasons, this approach should not merely involve the criminalization of these harmful practices.

It is not just that genital cutting practices are too common to practically enforce their criminalization in many places. More significantly, it is that criminal laws against female genital mutilation are almost always unenforced in developed countries where only a minority of a minority practice it. For example, every state and territory in Australia criminalized female genital mutilation decades ago, yet to date there has been only one successful prosecution, and it hinged on a guilty plea. There are a few reasons for this. Many survivors of genital mutilation do not want their parents to have a criminal conviction or go to prison. They also understand that often their parents have suffered the same form of abuse, so they do not report their parents to authorities. And as a nurse I knew once told me, many health professionals and social workers recognize that reporting female genital mutilation could result in children being taken away from their parents, and they weigh that against the potential for future harm being minimal given the procedure has already been performed. Aside from a lack of reporting, because of a fallible trial system, a significant imbalance of resources between the State and individual defendants, and the significant penalties associated with criminal offences, the prosecution rightly bears a high burden of proof, with guilt needing to be proven beyond a reasonable doubt and a presumption of innocence being fundamental principles of the criminal justice system. While entirely appropriate, this can make successful criminal prosecutions difficult.

What is needed to tackle non-consensual, medically unnecessary alterations of people's bodies is a mix of civil and criminal laws, an administrative mechanism for distinguishing between medically permissible and prohibited procedures, a focus on restorative justice, a complaints-based civil regulatory scheme that adopts a human rights-based approach, and redress and support for survivors of these practices. In addition, community education and awareness campaigns about the harms of genital cutting and details of newly implemented laws and regulations are required.

Whatever legislative and regulatory model jurisdictions adopt, many will likely provide religious exemptions for circumcision of the penis, because even in developed countries where these laws and regulations are more likely to pass, there remain large religious minorities with powerful lobbies. The silver lining is that even with religious exemptions, such laws, if they are formulated well, will protect most boys in developed countries where religious groups that practice male genital cutting account for the minority of such procedures.[65]

Recall that South Africa is an example of a country that has introduced legislation with such exemptions, in that it prohibits the circumcision of males under age 16 unless for religious or medical reasons. Most of the South African population is Christian, so what is more significant in rendering this legislation ineffectual is the broad medical exemption. Essential to the success of any legislation outlawing non-consensual, medically unnecessary alterations of people's bodies will be that it clearly defines and establishes "medical necessity" as the test by which medical interventions can be performed when an individual's own informed consent is unable to be obtained.[66]

...

Children are people, not property. Parents do not have a right to cut off parts of their children's bodies, nor to have someone else do it for them. All medically unnecessary genital cutting, including religious genital cutting, should be postponed until children are old enough to provide their own informed consent to the permanent removal of a part of their body. This simple proposition seems straightforward enough, but it is complicated by what many religious parents perceive as their religious duty to cut their children at a certain age: religious Jews circumcise their sons strictly on the eighth day after birth, whereas Muslim boys are often cut anywhere from several days to several years old. This and other differences between genital cutting in Judaism and Islam, as well as how despite their differences Jews and Muslims came to revere the same practice of male genital cutting, and how Christians came to be ambivalent about it, will be explored throughout the next chapter.

8

A religious rite that's wrong

Genital cutting practices predate monotheistic religion and indeed recorded history. As such no one is certain of how or why these practices first originated, but how they came to be practiced or rejected by followers of the three Abrahamic religions of Judaism, Christianity and Islam is much clearer.

Circumcision in Judaism

Female genital mutilation has never been widely practiced or permitted by the Jewish people,[1] the only notable exception being Ethiopian Jews, who performed various types of female genital mutilation for cultural rather than religious reasons,[2] but who largely abandoned the practice after their mass emigration to Israel in the late twentieth century.[3] As for male circumcision, there's evidence indicating it was a common practice in the Arabian Peninsula as far back as 4000 BCE, when two peoples migrated to what is now known as Iraq. Those two groups were the Sumerians and the Semites, the latter of which were the forefathers of the Hebrews. Whatever the reasons for its origination, within Judaism male circumcision came to represent a covenant, detailed in Genesis Chapter 17, between God and a ninety-nine-year-old shepherd called Abram, whose name God changed to Abraham.[4] God also changed Abraham's eighty-nine-year-old wife's name from Sarai to Sarah, and promised to bless her with the joy of geriatric childbirth,[5] despite this being physically impossible for Sarah; not to mention the improbability of ninety-nine-year-old Abraham rising to the occasion.

In this covenant, God plays a celestial real estate agent and power broker, promising Abraham and his descendants land, and that Abraham will be the "father of a multitude of nations."[6] In return, God asks for the genital cutting of all Abraham's male descendants in perpetuity,[7] adding that boys should be circumcised at eight days old, and that any Jewish male who is not circumcised is spiritually cut off from God, the Jewish people, and has broken the covenant.[8] As a sign of the times, and God's apparent indifference to slavery, there's also an admonishment that "He who is eight days old shall be circumcised among you, every male throughout your generations, he who is born in the house, or bought with money from any foreigner who is not of your offspring."[9] Modern-day readers are no doubt the sort of people who reject slavery, so any that still revere the immediately preceding words in the very same sentence that tell them to circumcise their sons might find it worthwhile asking themselves why.

Modern-day Jews abhor slavery as much as anyone else, yet most still see nothing wrong with cutting off their sons' foreskins, and Genesis 17 serves as the scriptural justification for doing so. It appears most are also unaware that despite being the first text in the Torah to mention circumcision, Genesis 17 was one of the last texts to be written. Indeed, Genesis 17, along with much of the rest of Genesis, much of Exodus and Numbers, and nearly all of Leviticus, was composed by the ruling rabbinic priestly class of the sixth century BCE. All these texts, along with Deuteronomy, were then compiled into a single Torah in the fifth century BCE.[10] Interesting timing, because biblical scholars estimate Abraham lived around 2100 and 1900 BCE.[11] Given the central importance the covenant in Genesis 17 is supposed to have, it's somewhat surprising it took well over a millennium for someone to write it down.

Perhaps even more surprising is that some scholars argue Moses – who it is written in Exodus led the Jewish people out of Egypt – originally rejected circumcision because he thought it to be only an Egyptian practice.[12] Again, given how central circumcision is supposed to be to Judaism, you'd think God would've taken a moment to explain this to Moses when talking to him through a burning bush, or in between the many plagues he is said to have tormented the Egyptians with. Yet God doesn't mention to Moses that circumcision is a requirement for the male descendants of Abraham until Leviticus 12. Interesting timing again, because the book and events of Leviticus come after Exodus, and we're told in Exodus that despite God not yet having informed Moses of the central importance of circumcision, God decided he ought to kill Moses for not being circumcised the Jewish way: "On the way at a lodging place, Yahweh [God] met Moses and wanted to kill him."[13] We're further told Moses was only saved by the quick thinking of his wife Zipporah, who "took a flint, and cut off the foreskin of her son, and cast it at his feet; and she said, "Surely you are a bridegroom of blood to me." So he [God] let him [Moses] alone. Then she [Zipporah] said, "You are a bridegroom of blood," because of the circumcision."[14]

Through Zipporah, Moses realised there is an Israelite method of circumcision distinct from the Egyptian (from examinations of mummified corpses it is known Egyptians performed only a dorsal slit of the foreskin). This difference is why God later commanded Moses' successor Joshua to "make flint knives, and circumcise again the sons of Israel [who had been circumcised in the Egyptian manner, to be circumcised for] the second time."[15] This second circumcision was in the Israelite manner – the full excision of the foreskin. One suspects that to many the Egyptian practice suddenly wasn't looking so bad by comparison.

This account of God almost murdering Moses and demanding the Israelites be "properly" circumcised could be taken to highlight how important circumcision is to God, and yet there are many intact Jewish men living full lives today, who aren't struck down by some almighty hand from the sky. It's as if God doesn't exist or doesn't care if Jewish men are circumcised or not. As for Moses, he certainly didn't exist, because as has now been proven – as fate would have it, by Jewish archaeologists – the events of Exodus never happened. The story of Exodus is a fiction based on thirteenth century BCE stories, penned sometime between the eighth and seventh centuries BCE, and refined in the sixth and fifth centuries BCE by the same rabbinic ruling class that inserted Genesis 17.[16] That's some bad news for religiously-minded Jews, because the story of Exodus is Judaism's primary historical narrative, but some good news for the ancient Egyptians, as God's alleged assault on their civilization and mass murder of their children turns out to also be fictitious.

If you think the events of Genesis, like Exodus, are nothing but a work of fiction, then you aren't alone, but it's understandable how Jewish parents who truly believe that the covenant between their people and God exists, and that its being broken has negative consequences, think the best thing they can do for their baby boy is to circumcise him. I also understand that many Jewish parents consider the failure to circumcise their sons means that they have themselves broken the covenant, rather than that they have merely broken it on behalf of their son. That's a difficult problem to get around. I can only acknowledge this impasse exists and reaffirm that the rights of children should take precedence given it is their bodies on the chopping block.

Clearly, any covenant cannot be freely entered into if the circumcision is performed on boys too young to consent to it. Surely a covenant agreed to by a consenting young man who understands the risks and religious implications is stronger than a covenant without the consent of an individual who understands neither. There's also no way of knowing if children will want to be party to this covenant with God, or that they will even believe in the God of Abraham, or any god, when they grow up. Parents who circumcise their children on religious grounds are violating their child's right to freedom of religion to indoctrinate them into their religion, yet they must realize it in no way guarantees their child's commitment to their religion. Indeed, I've spoken to Jewish atheists who said it was reflecting on the fact they were circumcised that first made them question their religious beliefs. They asked why God, who made them this way, would want them to change. They also asked why God would base a covenant around something as perverse as the cutting of children's genitals. They're fair questions. The answer many have come to is that no such god exists, that religion is merely the product of a superstitious pattern-seeking species of ape, and that the tale of the covenant with Abraham is just one of their many fables.

What's notable about Jewish atheists having jettisoned their belief in God is that it hasn't diminished their Jewish identity. Though belief in God is gone, a proud culture remains, because Jewish identity needn't be tied with belief in God, just as it needn't be tied with circumcision. Yet, curiously, I have met Jewish atheists who still had their boys circumcised. It would seem religious beliefs are easier to cast aside than cultural traditions, which often happen to include religious practices.[17] Given the steadfastness with which even irreligious Jews hold to their traditions in general, and the tradition of male circumcision in particular, it is worth considering exactly what this tradition entails.

The Jewish circumcision ceremony is called the *bris*, or *brit milah* (*brit* meaning covenant and *milah* meaning circumcision). I've already mentioned that Jewish circumcision involves the excision of the entire foreskin, but this wasn't always the case. Originally, *milah* entailed only the removal of the tip of the foreskin overhanging the head of the flaccid penis. Then, to stop Jewish men from stretching what was left of the foreskin to restore it, came *peri'ah* – the ripping of the fused foreskin from the head of the penis, and cutting all of it off so the entire head of the penis remains exposed.[18] This is the type of circumcision most people in the developed world are familiar with. I suspect, however, that most people would be less familiar with the traditional Jewish circumcision practice of *metzitzah b'peh*, in which the person who performs the circumcision, known as a mohel, sucks the bleeding wound of the penis and spits out the blood. I also suspect they'd be surprised to know this remains a common practice in the ultra-Orthodox Jewish community today. In New York City, for example, tens of thousands of infant boys have been subjected to this dangerous practice since the turn of the new millennium, and over a dozen babies have reportedly contracted herpes simplex virus type 1 (HSV-1),[19] of which at least two have been left with serious brain damage and another two have died as a result of the virus entering their bloodstream when their penises were sucked by infected mohels.[20]

Their deaths are made all the more tragic because the very reason for the existence of the practice of *metzitzah b'peh* is that rabbinical literature written in the fifth century CE argues it is dangerous *not* to suck the bleeding wound.[21] You'd expect this kind of thinking from people who didn't know microbes exist, but that it has persisted to the present day – long after the advent of modern medicine and an established germ theory of disease – is testament not just to how tightly the religious cling to their traditions, but to the obscenities the rest of us are willing to tolerate so they don't have to let go.

We have health and safety regulations for a reason – they stop people dying, provided you apply them. The response of New York City Mayor Bloomberg's administration to infants left brain-damaged or dead because of a herpes infection from *metzitzah b'peh* was merely to require mohels to have parents sign a consent form.[22] Pathetically unobtrusive as this measure was, mohels still refused to use the consent forms, citing religious freedom as their excuse. The de Blasio administration proved even more spineless when it abandoned the consent forms in 2015.[23] The failure of health authorities in New York to ban *metzitzah b'peh*, or at the very least to ban herpes-infected mohels from performing it, is frankly unforgivable.

Fortunately, despite its popularity in some places like New York, *metzitzah b'peh* remains a minority practice in Judaism; and the day the practice becomes a historical one can't come soon enough. In the meantime, the use of sterile glass tubes by some mohels to reduce the risk of infection when sucking the blood from the bleeding penile wound represents progress of a kind.

Despite male circumcision, and the yet more perverse practice of *metzitzah b'peh* having persisted into the twenty-first century, in what one might also call progress of a kind, due to its symbolic cutting and spilling of blood, it is thought by some scholars that ritual circumcision became a substitute for child sacrifice.[24] This I think is the only good thing to be said of it.

It has also been suggested that circumcision originated because it was believed to promote fertility, as does pruning a fruit tree;[25] a belief which somehow persisted despite foreskins not growing back as pruned branches do. As an explanation for male circumcision's ubiquity in Jewish culture, however, the desire to enhance fertility seems a rather weak one. A stronger explanation is that obligatory Jewish male circumcision originated as a rite of initiation in a male-dominated society.

In his book, *Marked in Your Flesh: Circumcision from Ancient Judaea to Modern America*, the cultural anthropologist Leonard Glick begins by expounding upon the origins of male circumcision as a distinctly Jewish practice, arguing this rite of initiation was as much for the father – who at the time was the one who performed the circumcision on his son, and bore the risk of his son's mutilation or death – as it was for the son himself. This rite of initiation was established and enforced by the rabbinic class that rose to prominence after a return from Babylonian exile; the same rabbinic class that in 516 BCE rebuilt the Second Temple from the ruins of the Jerusalem Temple, earlier destroyed by the Babylonians in 586 BCE; and that authored references to circumcision in Genesis 17 and Leviticus 12, because their new social order required a pact sealed with blood. As Glick put it, the rabbinic class sought "to maintain an ethnically exclusive patriarchy, dedicated to worship of Yahweh [God], and committed to sexual and marital restrictions to prevent reproductive contamination. What better way to accomplish this than by requiring that every male child be indelibly marked at birth?"[26]

As if the sanctification of genital cutting to be part of some ethnically exclusive boys' club wasn't repellent enough, it turns out the reason for it being performed at eight days old was also overtly misogynistic. Aside from Genesis 17, the only other time circumcision is mentioned as a requirement in the Torah is in Leviticus 12, when God instructs Moses and the Israelites on how to treat women after childbirth:

> *[God] spoke to Moses, saying, "Speak to the children of Israel, saying, 'If a woman conceives, and bears a male child, then she shall be unclean seven days; as in the days of her monthly period she shall be unclean. In the eighth day the flesh of his foreskin shall be circumcised. She shall continue in the blood of purification thirty-three days. She shall not touch any holy thing, nor come into the sanctuary, until the days of her purifying are completed. But if she bears a female child, then she shall be unclean two weeks, as in her period; and she shall continue in the blood of purification sixty-six days.*[27]

So, there you have it. Ritually, as determined by the priesthood, circumcision was performed on boys at eight days old because they'd been in contact with their mothers' blood, and so were believed to be impure for the first seven days following childbirth. Also note the way women who gave birth to a girl were treated as being doubly impure. One wonders what was done when a twin boy and girl were born. Was the boy's circumcision performed at 15 rather than 8 days old in such cases? Whatever the answer to this question was back in the day, it's no longer relevant to modern-day Jews, because purity in the context of Leviticus 12 related to maintaining the sanctity of the Second Temple, and this lost all practical application when it was destroyed in 70 CE by the Romans.[28] Yet long after the destruction of the Second Temple, Jewish circumcision has continued to be performed on the eighth day due to the explicit requirement as set out in Genesis 17, even though it was written by the same priestly class that authored the purity rules regarding circumcision in Leviticus 12, and so presumably mentioned the need for circumcision being performed on the eighth day in Genesis 17 for the same reason. In both Genesis 17 and Leviticus 12 we're told it is God who says that circumcision is to be performed on the eighth day, which leads one to ask, if the reason provided for circumcision being performed on the eighth day in Leviticus 12 is no longer relevant, why is reference to the eighth day in Genesis 17 still relevant? The answer appears to be that many consider the covenant in Genesis 17 to be a separate matter to the purity rules, despite the fact no reason is provided in Genesis 17 for circumcision needing to be performed on the eighth day.

The medieval Jewish philosopher and physician Moses Maimonides (1135–1204 CE) argued that circumcisions must be performed on the eighth day after birth because he believed all living things were weak in the first seven days of life, and that only from the eighth day after birth can they "enjoy the light of the world."[29] Whatever that is supposed to mean. Certainly, many doctors who perform circumcisions are content to do so within the first few days after birth. Infants aren't too weak for the procedure, just too weak to defend themselves from it being forced upon them.

Speaking more generally (and coherently), Maimonides wrote that circumcision must be performed on young boys for three reasons: 1) left to grow up, they might not submit to be circumcised; 2) young children do not feel much pain due to weak imaginations, whereas adults suffer from the premonition of pain; and 3) parents do not care much for their young children.[30] My level of disagreement with Maimonides on these three points is about the level of my eyebrows when I first read them. First, the deliberate violation of a child's future self-interest and autonomy does not justify the present violation of their bodily integrity. Most children who are not forcibly circumcised do not choose to be later in life, so they are not only robbed of making a choice, but of making the choice they in all probability would have made given the freedom to do so. Second, while infants cannot suffer from the premonition of pain, it is simply not the case that infants feel less physical pain than older children and adults, as both their screams during circumcision and the medical evidence attest to. Third, I have never met a parent who wasn't most in love with their child in its infancy. In fact, I have it on good authority from every parent who has ever raised a teenager that Maimonides has this one backwards. I joke of course. I can understand how parents living at a time when they could expect most children to die during infancy might not let themselves get so attached to their young children. In a time of low infant mortality, however, this last point seems both heartless and wrong.

Maimonides also spoke very plainly of the reasons for circumcision being the dulling of sexual pleasure and desire and the moderation of man by weakening the "organ of generation" as far as possible.[31] According to Maimonides, there can be no doubt that circumcision weakens sexual excitement.[32] Maimonides was not only concerned with reducing male pleasure, however, for he also noted it is difficult for women who have slept with intact men to separate from them, which according to Maimonides is the best reason to circumcise.[33] Reducing future sexual enjoyment probably doesn't strike you as sufficient reason to justify hacking away at a child's genitals, yet according to Maimonides it is the best reason for doing so. And Maimonides wasn't alone in thinking this. As we examined earlier, several hundred years after Maimonides last drew breath, this same medieval justification for genital cutting was employed in a failed effort to stop boys masturbating.

No doubt many Jewish readers thought to themselves just how outdated reference to Maimonides is. Some rabbis have stated as much publicly. For example, Rabbi Harold Kushner has said to "forget Maimonides … because on issues of sexuality Maimonides has some very medieval ideas."[34] Maimonides' ideas on sexuality were indeed medieval, so anyone who says to forget Maimonides might want to also consider forgetting circumcision.

Compared to other religions, Judaism has historically been good at adapting to changing times and new information, and arguably this has not diminished Jewish identity, but strengthened it. Abandoning circumcision need not be seen as a break from tradition, identity, or belonging, but rather as a continuation and progression of it. In fact, there is a growing pro-intact Jewish movement,[35] and at its helm are groups like Bruchim and Beyond the Bris, which welcome non-circumcising Jews and celebrate *brit shalom*, a ceremony that unlike *brit milah* does not entail circumcision. And, as Lisa Braver Moss, author of *A Measure of his Grief*, a novel about circumcision, has said, in her experience it is rare that a fellow Jewish person would not welcome non-circumcising families to their congregation.[36]

So why are Jewish people increasingly leaving their sons intact? The answer, I believe, is that circumcision in Judaism has its roots in the patriarchal, misogynistic teachings of theocratic zealots obsessed with sexual and ethnic purity, and many modern-day Jews see absolutely no reason to continue the bizarre practices of a cult like theirs.

Circumcision in Christianity

Given Jesus was Jewish, as were the original Christians, you might wonder how the Jewish practice of circumcision fell by the wayside in Christianity. It turns out the apostles who spread Jesus' teachings after his death are to thank for this, as they decided at the first council meeting of apostles and elders in Christian history that circumcision was not obligatory. The meeting was held in Jerusalem and was precipitated by an event that triggered shock waves among the early Christian Jews. It all started with a Roman centurion called Cornelius, who it is said invited the apostle Peter to his house following a vision.[37] As a Jew, Peter was not allowed to enter a pagan's house, but we are told Peter had a vision of his own which caused him to break the rules. It is said during Peter's vision a voice told him to eat food Jews considered unclean. Peter initially refused to eat the food, but the voice repeated, "What God has cleansed, you must not call unclean."[38] The voice then spoke to Peter again, telling him to go with the men sent by Cornelius the centurion to retrieve him.[39] Peter went with them, and later baptized the centurion and those in his household.[40]

The early followers of Jesus questioned Peter's actions, asking him why he ate with uncircumcised men.[41] In his defense, Peter told them about his vision, and so the council meeting of apostles and elders was called in Jerusalem.[42] The conclusion of the council was that circumcision is not obligatory, with the apostle James saying they should not trouble Gentiles who turn to God, but rather encourage them to "abstain from the pollution of idols, from sexual immorality, from what is strangled, and from blood."[43] This reading has also been interpreted as an abolition of the purity rules and a lifting of the prohibition against eating pork, so in addition to not missing out on foreskins, Christians can thank the apostle James for not missing out on bacon.

After the council meeting the apostles went about seeking converts for their new religion. The apostle Paul was one of the apostles charged with converting pagans, many of whom found circumcision barbaric, and would've been restricted by laws against circumcision and other Jewish practices even if they were partial to the idea of taking a sharp instrument to their genitals. This is the context in which Paul sought converts, so it isn't surprising that when writing to Titus he said there are "many unruly men, vain talkers and deceivers, especially those of the circumcision, whose mouths must be stopped: men who overthrow whole houses, teaching things which they ought not, for dishonest gain's sake."[44] Not one to mince words, Paul also said, "Beware of the dogs; beware of the evil workers; beware of the false circumcision."[45] The irony of calling Jews dogs would not have been lost on Paul, for it was common for Jews to refer to non-Jews in this manner; even Jesus is said to have done so.[46]

One can broadly, and with great simplification, describe the early followers of Jesus as belonging to one of two camps: a group of Jewish origin mainly known as the Nazarenes, and a group of pagan origin that would later come to be called the Christians, the latter of which was led by Paul. In the end it was Paul's group that won the day, in large part thanks to the decision of the Council of Jerusalem that circumcision need not be obligatory. Whether the early followers of Jesus rejected circumcision as an obligatory practice based on purported visions, a pragmatic approach to gaining converts, or both, what is clear is that concern for bodily autonomy and integrity did not inform their stance.

The consequence of the Council of Jerusalem prioritizing Peter's visions and Paul's proselytizing over a genuine concern for human wellbeing is that, as one might expect when a practice is not prohibited, but rather simply not obligatory, some Christians continued to circumcise, most notably Coptic Christians. Throughout history, however, circumcision has been denounced by Christian clerics. For example, the 11th session of the Ecumenical Council of Florence in 1442 CE firmly rejected circumcision, stating in no uncertain terms that, "[It] strictly orders all who glory in the name of Christian, not to practise circumcision either before or after baptism, since whether or not they place their hope in it, it cannot possibly be observed without loss of eternal salvation."[47] Of course, their rejection of the distinctly Jewish practice of circumcision isn't surprising given how rampant antisemitism was among most Christians at the time, and it remained rampant until well into the twentieth century. It wasn't until almost two thousand years of Jew-hating and branding of Jews as Christ killers had contributed to the extermination of several million Jewish people in the Holocaust[48] that Pope Paul VI finally (though even then still controversially), in 1965, declared in his *Nostra Aetate* that Jews were no more responsible for the death of Jesus than Christians.[49]

The *Nostra Aetate* has also given rise to the general view among Catholic clergy, as explained in 2002 by Cardinal Walter Kasper (then president of the Holy See's Commission for Religious Relations with Jewry), that Jewish people do not need to convert to Christianity in order to obtain eternal salvation.[50] Though flagrant antisemitism is thankfully no longer promoted by the Catholic Church, a general opposition to circumcision remains, as evidenced by a speech Pope Benedict XVI gave in 2007, in which he reminded the faithful that the Catholic Church is "a Church without circumcision" thanks to the Council of Jerusalem, following which circumcision ceased to be part of the Christian identity, with Christians being considered children of Abraham simply through their faith in Christ.[51]

The Catholic Church's popular opposition to circumcision goes beyond a speech by one of its least popular popes. Under the heading "respect for bodily integrity" the Catholic Church's catechism[52] no. 2297 states that "except when performed for strictly therapeutic medical reasons, directly intended amputations, mutilations, and sterilizations performed on innocent persons are against the moral law."[53] Unfortunately for the thousands of boys who were castrated for church choirs from the mid-sixteenth to late nineteenth centuries, the catechisms of the Catholic Church were not published until 1994, although fortunately for many others it did not take this long for the practice of castration to be abandoned.[54]

Despite the Catholic Church's clear opposition to circumcision, there remain evangelical Christians from various other denominations who, based on their reading of Genesis 17, circumcise in the belief it will bring them closer to God. And Christians of all stripes had no qualms accepting male circumcision as a means of preventing masturbation in the late nineteenth century. Although this reason for circumcision has long since been forgotten or remains unknown to most people, the widespread popularity of circumcision that resulted from it has led many (particularly American) Christians to blindly accept male circumcision as normal.

The tradition of genital cutting extends much further back in time for Coptic Christians in Egypt, who continue to cut the genitals not just of boys, but also girls. Like other Christians, Copts recognize male circumcision as something that is not necessary to the faith, and which shouldn't be done after baptism, but they nonetheless continue to circumcise their sons for reasons of hygiene and tradition.[55] And despite the protestations of Coptic religious authorities, who generally oppose female genital mutilation, many Egyptian Copts continue to cut their girls for reasons of chastity and marital eligibility.[56]

Circumcision in Islam

We've seen that Christians, with the notable exception of some evangelicals, generally don't cut their children's genitals for religious reasons, but that many Jewish parents do when it comes to boys. However, the number of boys circumcised by Jews is a drop in the ocean compared to the number circumcised by Muslims. This is to be expected, given that at the time of writing there are roughly 15 million Jews and 1.9 billion Muslims globally. Indeed, Muslims account for 70% of all circumcised males.[57]

The Arabic word for female circumcision is *khafd*, and the word for male circumcision is *khitan*,[58] the syllables of which (*kh-t-n*) pertain to primitive Semitic language, highlighting the fact that circumcision was an Arab custom predating Islam.[59] Indeed, as we've already seen, there's no doubt genital cutting long predates Islam, because it predates Judaism, which predates Islam. Of course, the fact genital cutting predates Islam doesn't mean it couldn't have been incorporated into the religion, as it was in the case of Judaism. Nonetheless, the argument that Islam mandates genital cutting turns out to be a tenuous one: circumcision is not mentioned once in the Qur'an. However, many Muslims continue to claim the practice is done for religious reasons, and that religious freedom should allow them to continue it.

A study of women in Somalia, where the population is almost entirely Muslim, and female genital mutilation is almost universal, found a majority reported cutting girls for religious reasons.[60] Many also reported that they worried no one would want to marry their daughter if she wasn't cut.[61] In Sudan, many believe if the clitoris isn't cut off it will become larger than a penis, eventually growing as long as a goose's neck.[62] Clearly social factors and a lack of education are playing a role in perpetuating the practice, and perhaps misguided religious observance is too.

Importantly, even though some Muslims practice male and female genital cutting, the question remains as to whether there is really any support for genital cutting in Islam. In other words, one should acknowledge the distinction between a religion and the actions of individuals who identify with that religion. Indeed, even if most Muslims practiced female genital cutting, this still wouldn't mean it's condoned or recommended in Islam, because religions are based on canonical texts and proclamations made by religious authorities, not on the actions of lay believers, which may or may not be congruent with the religion itself.

Since it isn't mentioned in the Qur'an, the belief genital cutting is recommended in Islam boils down to only a few verses in the *hadith*, which are the recorded accounts of the statements and deeds of the religion's founder, Muhammad. Among other things, the hadith list different things as *fitra*, the meaning of which is something like "natural disposition" and relates to purity and being free from sin. Different hadith describe different things as being fitra, most of which relate to cleanliness and hygiene. Although some hadith mention circumcision as fitra,[63] alongside things like the clipping of nails and moustaches, and cutting of pubic and armpit hair, many hadith do not refer to circumcision as fitra at all.[64] If circumcision really is an important act of fitra, why is it so often not mentioned as being so? In hadith that do refer to circumcision as fitra, there is no indication as to whether this relates to males or females, which has led some to think it applies to both.

One of the most influential verses in perpetuating female genital mutilation belongs to a hadith in which it is said, "A woman used to perform circumcision in Medina. The Prophet [Muhammad] said to her: Do not cut severely as that is better for a woman and more desirable for a husband."[65] Despite its influence with lay Muslims, the authenticity of this hadith has been questioned and repudiated by several Islamic scholars.[66] Indeed, it is unlikely Muhammad would have spoken to a woman about such matters, much less spoken so candidly. But even if true, this verse does nothing to establish female genital cutting as a requirement in Islam. Although one could argue Muhammad tacitly condoned female genital mutilation, for he didn't oppose it outright, he certainly didn't prescribe female genital cutting and made a point of saying it should not be severe. One can extend this logic to say that the less severe the better, such that not performing any genital cutting at all is the best possible outcome.

Female genital mutilation is common in many parts of Africa, and its practice is not just limited to Muslims. In countries such as Egypt, Kenya, Nigeria, and Tanzania the practice of female genital mutilation continues to be popular among Muslims and Christians, despite many religious authorities opposing it. So, what's going on here? It could be that although female genital mutilation is not mandated by religion, many still consider it a religious obligation because sexual purity has a central focus in all monotheistic religions.[67]

In contrast to the prevalence of female genital cutting in African countries with large Muslim populations, in the Middle East most Muslims do not mutilate their daughters' genitals. Indeed, most Arab Muslims are shocked to learn that other Muslims practice female genital mutilation. There are of course exceptions. In the Arab world, female genital mutilation is relatively common in Yemen,[68] Saudi Arabia,[69] Iran,[70] and some Kurdish communities scattered throughout various Arab nations.[71] Female genital mutilation is also common in Asian Muslim-majority countries like Malaysia[72] and Indonesia,[73] and within minority Muslim populations such as the Malay Muslims in the south of Thailand,[74] Malay Muslims in Singapore,[75] Sheedi and Bohra Muslims in Pakistan,[76] and Bohra Muslims in India,[77] to name a few. With Muslim immigration, female genital mutilation has also found its way into many developed nations (including those that once allowed it for dubious medical reasons and have since outlawed it), which are now struggling to deal with the problem, with laws against female genital mutilation almost always unenforced. Given how widespread female genital mutilation is globally, it would seem the focus on Africa is unfounded, save for the fact more severe forms of cutting tend to be practiced there.

Despite the practice being so widespread, there is undoubtedly division among Muslims when it comes to the permissibility of female genital cutting, with most Muslims worldwide being opposed to it. Unfortunately, there is no such division when it comes to male genital cutting, as Muslims everywhere tend to favor it. Islam recognizes Abraham as a prophet, and it appears Muslims mainly circumcise their boys for reasons of tradition, ritual hygiene, and in certain cases as a rite of initiation into manhood, rather than in strict adherence to scripture, and certainly not as part of any covenant with God as is the case with Jews. Tradition and hygiene also influence the decision of Jewish parents to circumcise their sons but, unlike Muslims, their claim that the practice is central to the religion is well founded in scripture. As already noted, in the case of Islam, male genital cutting is not mentioned in the Qur'an, and much debate exists about whether it is clearly prescribed in the hadith, required for conversion, or should be regarded as obligatory or merely recommended, although at a minimum male circumcision is usually considered to be recommended.

This is in stark contrast to Judaism, which except in its most liberal branches requires circumcision of male converts and newborns for them to be considered Jewish in the religious sense of the word.

Other notable differences between male circumcision in Judaism and Islam are that: 1) as mentioned earlier, boys are circumcised at eight days old in Judaism, whereas Muslim parents circumcise their sons as early as seven days or as late as several years old, the timing of which is dependent on geography and local custom, and 2) Islamic male circumcision tends to only involve the partial removal of the foreskin, such that some of the head of the penis remains covered; although if the circumcision is performed by a doctor in the Anglosphere, Muslims are likely to have the full excision, as this has become the method of choice for Jews and throughout the developed world.

...

The genital cutting of children is justified in different places and to different degrees through a mix of social, cultural, and religious reasons. If we base our understanding of religions on their canonical texts, and the statements and actions of religious authorities, rather than those of lay believers, then: in Judaism, male circumcision is usually interpreted as obligatory for males and female genital mutilation is condemned. In Christianity, female genital mutilation is condemned, while male circumcision is not required but is nonetheless often done by Coptic Christians and sometimes done by evangelicals; and although condemnation of male circumcision was historically linked with antisemitism, modern-day opposition at least within the Catholic Church is linked with a growing concern about, and understanding of, bodily autonomy and human rights. In Islam, male circumcision is not obligatory, although it is usually recommended for reasons of ritual hygiene and tradition, whereas the genital cutting of females is widely debated by Islamic scholars, and the tide has turned in favor of those who argue it is not recommended in Islam. In the end, even if female genital cutting were mandated in Islam, as many say it is for males in Judaism, many already reject female genital mutilation and refuse to accept religious freedom as an excuse for it, so permitting the genital cutting of boys on religious grounds represents an indefensible double standard.

9

Not so clear cut

In the US, such is the degree of mistrust some parents have for the medical profession that they put ankle bands on their newborn boys that read, "Do not circumcise or retract."[1] The warning against retracting the foreskin is included because, as already noted, the newborn foreskin is fused to the head of the penis and should not be retracted. The admonishment against circumcision is also included because some parents fear their son might be circumcised without their consent. Their fears are not totally unfounded since, as the following examples show, circumcisions without parental consent in the US are not unheard of. In 1979, a one-month-old boy developed meningitis and subsequent brain damage two days after being circumcised without parental consent, resulting in a settlement of $1,000,000.[2] In 1992, a boy born at the Jackson Hospital and Clinic in Montgomery, Alabama, was circumcised without parental consent. The boy's parents sued and were awarded $65,000 in damages.[3] In 1997, a newborn boy was circumcised by an obstetrician at the Quincy Medical Center in Massachusetts, even though no parental consent form had been signed, and even though the parents had previously told the hospital they did not want their son circumcised, resulting in a total settlement payment of $115,000.[4]

Although consent is now more strictly sought for circumcisions in the US, there is still a long way to go for current medical practice in the US to catch up with standards in the rest of the developed world. According to Georganne Chapin, the founder of Intact America, "The only thing that is required for a doctor or midwife or other practitioner in a health care setting to circumcise a boy is for the parent (just one parent – usually the mother) to sign a consent form saying s/he has been informed about the procedure and the risks it entails."[5] It is problematic to say the least that consent is only required from one parent, but even more remarkably, it appears that even though consent is sought, very often it is not *informed* consent. Chapin has advised me Intact America has "talked with countless mothers who say that the consent form was included in a large packet of materials they were given when they registered at the hospital prior to giving birth; or that the consent form was first flashed in their face a few hours after childbirth by a doctor or nurse pushing circumcision, or simply assuming it was going to be done."[6] Worse still, the actions of many hospital staff appear coercive, Intact America hears "from many, many parents who say that they were asked four, five, six times by hospital staff (usually nurses) if they planned to circumcise, even after saying NO. [Intact America] have even heard from parents who were told they need to sign a form to "opt out" of circumcision – this is unheard of for any other (even medically indicated) procedure."[7]

Informed consent is the cornerstone of modern medical ethics. Wherever possible the informed consent of the patient is required, and invasive surgical procedures should not be performed on children too young to consent when the procedures are not medically necessary. As the British Medical Association detailed in a statement offering guidance for doctors on male circumcision, it is unethical and inappropriate to circumcise, even for therapeutic reasons, when other techniques are at least as effective and less invasive.[8] In other words, that circumcision is sometimes therapeutic is not a sufficient justification for it. However, simply being more therapeutic than other treatment options still doesn't make circumcision an ethical choice when performed on minors too young to provide informed consent. If the treatment is not urgent, and by virtue of not being urgent, not medically necessary, then it remains unethical to perform circumcision on a child who is too young to consent, because the procedure could be deferred until they are old enough to provide consent.

Even with "parental consent", routine infant circumcision remains unethical, because as with all unnecessary surgeries, it is only the consent of the person going under the knife that matters. The fact infants cannot consent to unnecessary surgery does not mean the right to consent is transferred to their parents. Rather, it means that the unnecessary surgery should be deferred until children are old enough to consent to it themselves. Of course, many proponents of circumcision are fully aware that if the choice were left to the individuals concerned, the majority would decide not to circumcise, and incredibly this is still used as an excuse for performing circumcision on infants when they are powerless to resist.

...

Violating someone's bodily autonomy is only morally permissible when the rights of other members of society collectively trump the rights of the individual. This exception to the rule is made when an individual poses harm to others. As the nineteenth-century English philosopher John Stuart Mill said in *On Liberty*, "the only purpose for which power can be rightfully exercised over any member of a civilized community, against his will, is to prevent harm to others. His own good, either physical or moral, is not a sufficient warrant ... Over himself, over his body and mind, the individual is sovereign."[9]

There are some who view routine infant circumcision of males as just such an example of a group's rights trumping an individual's rights. They cite the potential for male circumcision to reduce sexually transmissible infections, and argue that since circumcision offers protection against certain infections, it should be supported for its public health benefits in the same way as routine child vaccination.[10] This is a rather sinister false equivalence, used to exploit the positive connotations associated with vaccination, which the overwhelming medical consensus is in support of, to endorse a surgical procedure that has many negative effects, and which the overwhelming medical consensus is opposed to. It also misleadingly suggests that routine infant male circumcision and routine child vaccination are equivalent in terms of their ability to reduce the spread of infection. They aren't. Unlike the benefits of vaccination, which are well established and accepted by the medical community, the claim that male circumcision reduces the transmission of HIV or other sexually transmissible infections is highly contested and debated by the medical community. But even *if* it were true that circumcision reduces the risk of some diseases, the comparison to vaccination is still false, because not only is vaccination far more effective, it also poses far fewer risks, and does not involve the permanent amputation of healthy tissue and the loss of its associated functions.

On different cultures

In many tribes and cultures, individuals are expected to go through certain rites of passage to be considered, or to remain part of, the group. Circumcision is one such rite of passage. In his autobiography, *Long Walk to Freedom*, Nelson Mandela described his own ritual circumcision at the age of 16 among the Xhosa, which marked his becoming a man.[11] In the Xhosa tradition, intact men are still considered to be boys, and they cannot marry or inherit the wealth of their fathers.[12] The lengthy and elaborate circumcision ritual Mandela describes involves a "daring exploit" in the days before the circumcision, which in his case involved stealing and slaughtering a pig, followed by singing and dancing the night before, and bathing in the river at dawn for "purification" before the circumcision.[13] During the circumcision itself, the boys are not allowed to flinch or cry for, as Mandela explained, to do so is a sign of weakness. Instead, boys must "suffer in silence" because "a boy may cry; a man conceals his pain."[14] And indeed, as they are cut without anesthetic, the Xhosa boys shout out "Ndiyindoda!" meaning "I am a man!" The ritual continues even after the cut. The severed foreskins are tied to blankets the naked boys are wrapped in, and they retire to a smoke-filled hut to paint their bodies in white ocher (another symbol of purity), before burying their foreskins somewhere in the forest – a symbolic burying of their childhood, but also traditionally a practice thought to prevent wizards using the foreskins for evil purposes.[15] The boys remain in the huts until their wounds are healed, and they are not to be seen by women during this time. Once healed, the boys reemerge from their huts, wash off the white ocher in the river, cover themselves in red ocher, and have sex with a woman, such that her body rubs off the red ocher; although as Mandela notes, in his case the red ocher "was removed with a mixture of fat and lard."[16]

How can we make sense of such an elaborate a ritual? And what can we make of each boy having to shout "I am a man!" as his part of his manhood is cut off? The boys are male, no doubt, but such an exclamation doesn't refer to biological sex. It refers instead to gender. Whether in Xhosa culture or any other, a young male is not considered a "man" until he has displayed certain behaviors and attributes, though what exactly these are depends on the culture in which the male resides. For the Xhosa, it appears a boy is not a man until he has learned to suppress his feelings of pain and slept with a woman. While many other cultures are also guilty of promoting toxic forms of masculinity, I am surely not alone in thinking that in general it is healthier for boys to be taught to express their feelings rather than to bottle them up, and to treat women with respect rather than as sex objects; yet there are people who recoil from such expressions of ethical common sense as the one I have just made, because they think morality is relative to different cultures, and consequently reject the notion that anyone should criticize the practices of other cultures. These people are called moral relativists, and they are as wrong as some of the practices to which they turn a blind eye.

Moral relativism and genital cutting

Non-consensual, medically unnecessary genital cutting is unethical. Note this statement presents two different criteria for consideration (consent and medical necessity). Performing surgical genital alterations on someone without their consent violates their bodily autonomy, and such a violation is only considered ethical in the rare instances it serves the best interests of an individual who is unable to provide informed consent (in the case of circumcision because the individual is usually an infant or young child). This is where the medical consideration becomes relevant, because it's only in cases that circumcision is medically *necessary* that it is in the best interests of the individual, and therefore acceptable to circumcise them without their informed consent, assuming they're unable to provide it. Cases of medically necessary circumcision are, however, exceedingly rare, and fortunately most cases of medically necessary circumcision apply to adults, or mature minors who, unlike young boys, can provide informed consent. Unfortunately, most circumcisions are medically unnecessary and performed on children too young to consent. This has, in part, been enabled by people who think circumcision to be morally impermissible for themselves and their culture, but who nonetheless think other people and cultures should be allowed to practice it.

Moral relativists argue that people should tolerate practices foreign to their own culture, such as genital cutting, because they believe there is no objective means with which to judge people from other cultures who see nothing wrong with such practices. It's this kind of reasoning that led the renowned feminist Germaine Greer to dedicate an entire chapter in *The Whole Woman* to the mutilation of female bodies without once condemning female genital mutilation.[17] In fairness to Greer, she rightly pointed out the moral hypocrisy of Westerners who oppose female genital mutilation in other cultures, while supporting the genital mutilation of boys and even girls in their own. Her labeling of Western opposition to female genital mutilation in Africa as "an attack on cultural identity" likely wouldn't have been received so critically had she argued it was an attack worth making. Instead, Greer wrote that while she thinks we should support feminists fighting to end female genital mutilation in their own countries, we should not do so "to the point of refusing to consider the different priorities and cultural norms by which other women live."[18] Greer suggested that female genital mutilation could represent a means by which women assert control over their own bodies, similar to tattoos and piercings, and asked why, if a woman from a place like Ohio has a right to have her genitals surgically altered, a woman from a place like Somalia should not have the same right.[19] Here Greer makes a major misstep, and conflates the voluntary genital modifications of consenting adults with the involuntary genital mutilations of children. Most Somali women, indeed, most women worldwide, are not making the decision to have their genitals cut – quite the opposite – most have it forced on them when they are young girls. It shouldn't be this difficult to get a feminist to explicitly reject all non-consensual, medically unnecessary female genital cutting, and Greer's failure to do so is deeply unfortunate.

Why do so many otherwise intelligent and decent people accept cultural difference as an excuse for the abuse of children, particularly when it takes the form of genital cutting? To answer this question, we need to clear some philosophical brush. In doing so we will examine exactly what moral relativism is and why it fails as a meta-ethical theory. (Meta-ethics is the branch of philosophy concerned with the foundation of ethics and the nature of ethical statements.) As will become clear, if moral relativism doesn't make any sense, people are entirely justified in making moral judgments about other cultures in general, and of the genital mutilation of children in other cultures in particular.

On the failings of moral relativism

When asked if the glass of water (or wine as I prefer to imagine it) is half full or half empty, there has never any doubt in my mind as to the correct answer – it is both at the same time. Is it right to judge the optimist for thinking it half full, or the pessimist for thinking it half empty, given I approach the question from a different (realist) point of view? Of course it is. The mere existence of different beliefs about the nature of the glass of water does not preclude the existence of an objectively correct answer. The *fact* of the matter is that something cannot be half empty without also being half full at the same time, and just because the optimist and the pessimist think otherwise doesn't make them right.[20] As with the glass of water, people approach moral questions differently, but the existence of different answers to moral questions does not preclude the existence of an objectively correct one.[21] The mistaken belief that it does is called meta-ethical moral relativism.

It's worth taking a moment to see how meta-ethical moral relativism is different to other types of moral relativism, because they're often confused. Moral relativists contend that: 1) morality is relative to time, place and person (descriptive moral relativism); 2) moral questions admit of no objectively right or wrong answers (meta-ethical moral relativism); and 3) for this reason we ought not to judge, but in fact to tolerate, what we perceive as the immoral behavior of others (normative moral relativism).

Moral relativism is correct in the descriptive sense, but *only* in that sense. It doesn't logically follow that just because people hold to different truths that there exists no objective truth of the matter.[22]

Normative moral relativists argue we cannot judge other cultures because we lack the necessary understanding to do so, yet they often praise other cultures, which is itself a judgment, and praise is worthless unless it is rooted in some form of understanding.[23] The assumption made, though often unstated, is clear: it's okay to judge other cultures if you have nothing bad to say. This unspoken rule seemingly does not apply to your own culture, for moral relativists tend to be as critical of their own culture as they are praising of others.

Reflecting on your culture by comparing it to others is valuable. But if moral truth exists only within cultures, as moral relativists argue, why do they also recognize the benefit of such comparisons? The reason they do is because without reference to moral standards (including those of other cultures, which can be better), all moral progress is impossible. These standards change over time as we weave through the ethical maze, but always with the (often unacknowledged) view that there is an end to it. Whether or not we will find it is another matter. It helps to meet others as we navigate our way through the maze, if for no other reason than they can show us their way leads to a dead end. The relativist trap is to think that they, and everyone else in the maze – all of them going in different directions – know the right way. The question then is by what standards do moral relativists judge moral progress? If the standards are entirely culturally dependent, as moral relativists suggest, then they shouldn't require reference to other cultures at all. The reality, however, is that we've much to learn from each other.

In going through the exercise of comparing cultures, it is necessary to first define what "culture" means. This is problematic, because whichever way one chooses to define it, one cannot ignore that monocultures do not exist outside of agriculture. Even the most isolated culture, immune to influences from outside sources – and such isolation is exceedingly rare in our increasingly globalized world – is still subject to divisive forces within that lead to the formation of subcultures. The question then becomes, who decides what constitutes any given culture? Do moral truths not exist within cultures, but rather within subcultures, or the individuals they're comprised of? These are questions moral relativists must answer if they insist that moral truths only exist within cultures because differences exist between them, because differences also exist within them. Meta-ethical moral relativism, while accepting of differences between cultures, seems to wrongly assume uniformity within them.

If the majority is to decide what constitutes any given "culture", or what is or isn't moral, then we are reduced to mere conventionalism. In this manner any practice can be condoned. Is the stoning to death of adulterers morally wrong in one culture and morally right in another, simply because majority opinion of the practice varies from one place to another? We have entered dangerous territory. Morality is not a matter of consensus.

As a meta-ethical theory, moral relativism represents a thoroughly confused and dangerous view of morality: it reduces morality to majority rule, provides no clear way to judge moral progress, and problems with defining culture leave open the question of how exactly it can have any practical application.

Moral relativism also has several questionable normative implications: for all their talk of not passing judgment on other cultures, moral relativists still often make positive judgments of them, and the entailment of tolerance remains logically contradictory, as well as morally vacuous given it can be used to justify absolutely anything – as indeed it is used today to justify no lesser crime than the mutilation of defenseless children. Moral relativists are not as moral as they like to think they are.

Much remains to be said about what is morally right or wrong, but before we can even begin that discussion, we must acknowledge that objective moral truths exist. In doing so, we must be moral realists as much as we are realists about the half-filled glass of water.

Genital mutilation is objectively morally wrong

Many people once thought that the Earth was flat, and they could not have been more wrong. Whereas this misconception came from ignorance of the natural world, moral misconceptions often come from the mistaken belief morality is somehow removed from it altogether. This belief comes from an understanding of the distinction between *facts* (which are descriptive and relate to how things are) and *values* (which are prescriptive and relate to how things should be), and the subsequent belief that how things *are* does not necessarily have any bearing on how they *should* (or ought) to be. In other words, you cannot get an "ought" from an "is". Philosophers know this as the "is-ought problem", which was first described by David Hume in his *Treatise of Human Nature*.[24] The severing of "is" and "ought" is referred to as Hume's guillotine, but we needn't lose our heads over it if we have a goal in mind.

The fact-value distinction and the is-ought problem are intertwined, for whereas facts relate to what is, values relate to how we ought or ought not to behave. Morality is thus seen by some as being beyond the realm of scientific inquiry, which deals with matters of fact. And yet it remains the case that ethical sentences express propositions, some of which are true, and that are made true by objective features of the world, regardless of subjective opinion. Philosophers call this ethical naturalism. There is debate about what those objective features should be, but wellbeing seems to me to be the ideal culmination of what various schools of thought in Greek ethics, with their different focuses on pleasure, virtue, and flourishing, were building towards. It also avoids the trap of utilitarianism based on happiness or preference, because wellbeing relates to what is good regardless of what makes one happy, or what one prefers. For example, being vaccinated against a deadly disease might make you unhappy if you don't like needles, and if your phobia of needles is severe enough, or you wrongly believe vaccination is bad for you, then you may even prefer not to be vaccinated, but the fact of the matter is that unless you are one of the few people who have a severe reaction to the adjuvants used in vaccines, being vaccinated is good for your wellbeing and also public health, whether you know it or not. And if your *goal* is to protect or enhance wellbeing, then the *fact* vaccination provides immunity to deadly diseases clearly means you *ought* to vaccinate.

Morality is relative in the descriptive sense, but this doesn't mean it can't be studied objectively within the context of the wellbeing of conscious creatures. This remains true regardless of the debate about whether moral considerations are the sole domain of moral philosophy, or whether some kind of science of morality can exist.[25] While I think that science has nothing to say about why we ought to value wellbeing in the first place, I think it has everything to say about why we ought to use vaccines, or ought *not* to mutilate children – or why we ought to do or ought not to do any number of things – if we value wellbeing and make it our goal to promote it.[26]

That we should value the health and wellbeing of children is a value judgment most people agree with, and that we should protect the health and wellbeing of children is a goal most people agree we should strive for, yet many parents nonetheless diminish their children's wellbeing by mutilating their genitals. Parents do so either because they are unaware of the harm, or because they think any physical or psychological harm caused is minor compared to the social, spiritual, or religious benefits their children might gain as a result.

What's interesting is that the value judgment and goal of parents who support genital cutting, namely valuing and protecting the health and wellbeing of children, is precisely the same as that held by people who oppose genital mutilation, yet both have concluded they should behave in different (indeed opposite) ways based on what they understand to be the facts. It would seem, then, that even with the same goal, based on the same value judgment, that the "ought" of cutting behavior depends on the "is" of its known (or unknown) harms, and the relative weight of importance one attributes to various forms of harm, whether physical, psychological, social, spiritual, religious, or whatever else.

The debate over the science of morality is irrelevant to the conclusion that moral relativism suffers from several fundamental flaws, and so cannot be used to excuse genital mutilation in other cultures. It is also irrelevant to the conclusion that non-consensual, medically unnecessary genital cutting is objectively wrong within the context of an ethical framework that values and has protecting and promoting health and wellbeing as its goal. Morality being relative in the descriptive sense does not preclude it being studied objectively, such as in the context of the wellbeing of conscious creatures. The only question that remains is why we should value the wellbeing of conscious creatures in the first place. It's a perfectly valid question, but it remains secondary to the question of why we should *not* value the wellbeing of conscious creatures. In the absence of a rational answer to this latter question, I think it reasonable to take valuing the wellbeing of conscious creatures as axiomatic.

...

It is a mistake to equate not knowing everything with not knowing better. Whatever knowledge we possess, the basis of progress in general and of moral progress in particular must be the understanding there is room for improvement. Most people already accept that their culture is on the whole better than other cultures that existed in the past, so they should have no qualms in judging cultural practices that exist at present, but which belong in the past. If we value wellbeing, then the simple fact is that a culture in which the genitals of children are left intact is objectively better than one in which they are mutilated.

10

Toward the final cut

It is the twenty-first century, and we are still mutilating children's genitals. Fortunately, as I write these words, there are people all over the world fighting to protect and promote everyone's right to bodily integrity, so that all children can keep the genitals they were born with, and every baby is brought home whole. Perhaps having read this far you now wish to count yourself among them. If that is the case, then know that there are many ways you can contribute. For example, you can leave your children intact, urge others to do the same, or join the movement and volunteer your time or donate to an organization that is working to protect children from the harms of non-consensual, medically unnecessary genital cutting.

The movement to protect children from the harms of genital cutting is often referred to as the "genital autonomy" or "bodily integrity" movement. Some people in this movement refer to themselves as "intactivists", a portmanteau of "intact" and "activists".[1] Whatever label people assign to the movement or themselves, they come from varied backgrounds: they can be cut or intact; many are doctors, nurses, and other health professionals; others are lawyers, human rights advocates, or self-identified "regret parents"; they come from all political persuasions and religious beliefs, or lack thereof. What these people all have in common is they understand and work to educate others about the harms of non-consensual, medically unnecessary genital cutting practices, so that these practices one day come to an end.

In many ways the genital autonomy movement in the US owes its prominence to Marilyn Milos.[2] As a young nurse, Milos witnessed the circumcision of a baby boy and has been fighting against it ever since. In 1985, she led a group of other health professionals in founding the National Organization of Circumcision Information Resource Centers (NOCIRC), later known as Genital Autonomy America. Milos has dedicated much of her life to protecting children, and both she and NOCIRC were instrumental in organizing the first International Symposium on Circumcision in 1989 and have remained heavily involved in the many symposia on the subject that have taken place since.

Following the founding of NOCIRC, several other non-profit organizations were established in the US, including Intact America, Attorneys for the Rights of the Child, Doctors Opposing Circumcision, the National Organization to Halt the Abuse and Routine Mutilation of Males (NOHARMM), Bruchim, Beyond the Bris, and Catholics Against Circumcision. It is no surprise that there are so many groups opposed to circumcision in the US, given how common the practice is there. But the movement of people advocating for everyone's right to bodily integrity and genital autonomy is global, with groups including The Darbon Institute in Australia and New Zealand, 15 Square in the UK,[3] the Children's Health & Human Rights Partnership in Canada, and Intact Denmark, to name a few. These organizations exist to educate people about the harms of medically unnecessary genital cutting, because these practices will come to an end only when enough people understand that they are harmful.

I met Marilyn Milos and many other inspiring people when I presented at the 13th International Symposium on Genital Autonomy and Children's Rights at the University of Colorado in 2014. After my speech, I went out walking with some friendly people I had just met to see how they engaged in what they called "public education". I wanted to understand how they go about spreading their knowledge of the harms of genital cutting. None of them had a medical background, and I was curious to see how much they knew about the medical arguments for and against male circumcision. I was pleased to find that not only were they non-confrontational, but they were also very knowledgeable when it came to the medical arguments. Their approach was to walk around with informative, inoffensive signs and shirts, ignoring the glares and insults of some passersby, and speaking only to those who stopped to talk. Assuming an observational role, I stood back and watched as they worked to educate people wanting to learn.

I'll never forget the moment two of my new friends spoke to a young man who had stopped to say he was circumcised as a boy and wanted to know more about it. Like many men he had never really thought about it before. I watched as this poor man realized he had a perfectly healthy and normal part of his body taken from him without his consent for no good (medically necessary) reason. He learned that aside from this being a violation of his human rights, it had resulted in a penis that is less sensitive, and sex and masturbation that is less pleasurable than it otherwise would have been. He left that conversation in what can only be described as a state of shock. Hurt and confused, he sat on a bench staring into the distance. I can only imagine what he must have been thinking. It was then the group moved on to educate other people about circumcision, leaving this man alone with his thoughts. All this left me feeling terribly uneasy. This man had learned a lot from the conversation, and if education is the sole purpose of such activism, then it was a resounding success. But what concerned me was that no one involved in this process was a professional counselor, and this man was clearly left in need of one. It is tempting, then, with many millions of circumcised men in America alone, to simply ignore the problem, tell no one of the harms of circumcision, and to avoid turning old physical wounds into new psychological ones. And yet this is both practically impossible and morally unconscionable, for the truth always gets out, and it is surely wrong to hide the abuse of some to spare their feelings when doing so condemns countless others to suffer the same fate.

One of the people I was with that day was Jonathon Conte, a gay man from San Francisco. Conte was circumcised as an infant and was a vocal critic of the practice all his adult life. I was saddened to learn that on May 9, 2016, he died by suicide.[4] I cannot claim to have known him well enough to be certain what led him to end his life, but from our few discussions, from observing his online activism for two years, and from accounts by people who knew him much better than I did, it is without question that he suffered psychological trauma from having been a victim of genital mutilation. In 2017, a British man named Alex Hardy also died by suicide. His note made it clear he decided to end his life because of circumcision harms.[5]

As people increasingly become conscious of the harms of genital cutting, we must ensure there are appropriate supports in place for people who have experienced these harms. There is a clear and pressing need for mental health professionals that are trained to deal with the trauma of genital cutting. Far too many survivors of genital mutilation find themselves seeking support from mental health professionals who at best know nothing about the issue, and at worst disregard their trauma or re-traumatize them. Had appropriate support been in place, Jonathon Conte, Alex Hardy, and others like them, might still be alive today.

...

When it comes to male circumcision, new and expecting parents face a myriad of different opinions, from those of medical professionals, to those of family and friends, and even complete strangers. This barrage of well-intentioned, but often emotionally charged and not-so-well-informed opinions inevitably makes for some fraught decision-making. For parents I offer a reprieve: the circumcision decision needn't be such a difficult one for them to make, because in the presence of medical necessity it is essentially a decision made for them by circumstance, and in the absence of medical necessity it is a decision parents have no right to make for their children in the first place. That said, if circumcision remains a socially and legally permitted practice, parents will continue to decide whether to circumcise their children. I've written this book in part to help parents make an informed decision, and indeed I hope the right one.

It is a tragedy that so many parents have been misled to the point they have unwittingly harmed their children in this most personal and permanent of ways, as indeed many were also harmed themselves by their parents when they were children. This cycle of abuse will only be broken by widespread understanding of the physical and psychological harms, and the breaches of medical ethics and human rights, associated with non-consensual, medically unnecessary genital cutting. That many in the medical profession have not only allowed the genital mutilation of children to occur, but performed and profited from it, is frankly unforgiveable.

Nothing, not one's social or aesthetic preferences, or even the most sincerely held religious belief, is a license for child abuse, and it is difficult to think of a more glaring example of child abuse than restraining a child and cutting off part of their body. All children have a right to the bodies they are born with, and all non-consensual, medically unnecessary alterations of their bodies represent a clear breach of medical ethics and human rights that should not be tolerated by any person or society.

All the arguments invoked to support male circumcision – that it's more hygienic, has medical benefits, looks better, or should be permitted because of tradition, religion, or because a lot of people do it – are also commonly used to support "female circumcision" in many parts of the world. In the developed world, however, we've outlawed "female circumcision" and abandoned this euphemism, because we recognize the non-consensual, medically unnecessary genital cutting of girls for what it really is: female genital mutilation. There will come a day when we also view the non-consensual, medically unnecessary genital cutting of boys as mutilation, but for millions of boys that day won't come soon enough.

Notes

1. Cutting to the chase: an introduction

1 Freeman 2015.
2 Associated Press in Boynton Beach, Florida 2015.
3 Freeman 2014.
4 Kaplan 2015.
5 Davis 2001; Earp 2015a.
6 World Health Organization 2007.
7 18 U.S. Code §116. Female genital mutilation. Legal Information Institute https://www.law.cornell.edu/uscode/text/18/116
8 AHA Foundation.
9 Beres 2016.
10 Smith 2015.
11 Onyulo 2018.
12 Sex characteristics are the physical features relating to sex, including genitalia and other sexual and reproductive anatomy, chromosomes, hormones and secondary physical features emerging from puberty.
13 Sneppen and Thorup 2016. 181 boys out of on average 10,858 (1.66%–1.7%) needed some kind of foreskin surgery in 2014, but only 53 of these (44 initially + 9 later; 0.5%) were circumcised.
14 Aly 2013.
15 World Health Organization 2008, 3.
16 Hitchens 2005.
17 Foreskin Restoration Intactivist Network.
18 In principle, each of these arguments could apply to other genital cutting or altering practices as much as male circumcision, but in practice they are employed differently depending on the individual's sex characteristics and the social, cultural, and religious expectations of their parents and society at large.

2. Not just a little snip

1 Rhinehart 1999; Svoboda and Van Howe 2013.
2 Warren 2010, 77.
3 Kigozi et al., 2006; Werker, Terng and Kon 1998.
4 DeLaet 2009.
5 Earp 2014.
6 Ibid.
7 World Health Organization 2018.
8 This WHO description ignores the fact that the clitoris extends beneath the skin like an iceberg under water, so it is never *totally* removed.
9 Notably, the amount of tissue removed varies widely between communities that practice this type of female genital mutilation.
10 Type I, II and III also have a number of subtypes depending on the exact nature of the cutting.

11 World Health Organization 2008, 24.
12 Bishai et al., 2010.
13 World Health Organization 2016.
14 Nocirc 2011.
15 Volksbegehren gegen Kirchen-Privilegien 2012.
16 I refer to 'avoidable' harm to a child because one can imagine unavoidable circumstances in which a child needs to undergo a painful but medically necessary procedure.
17 American Academy of Pediatrics Committee on Bioethics 2010, 1092.
18 Moldwin and Valderrama 1989; Winkelmann 1956.
19 Cold and Taylor 1999, 41.
20 Cold and Taylor 1999.
21 Richters, Gerofi, and Donovan 1995; Van Duyn and Warr 1962.
22 Taves 2002.
23 Bensley and Boyle 2003; Frisch, Lindholm, and Grønbæk 2011; O'Hara and O'Hara 1999.
24 Iwasaki 2010.
25 Cold and Taylor 1999.
26 Camille, Kuo, and Wiener 2002; Cold and Taylor 1999.
27 Gairdner 1949; Kayaba et al., 1996; Oster 1968.
28 Camille, Kuo, and Wiener 2002.
29 Iwasaki 2010.
30 A study to determine what advice was given to Utah mothers by pediatricians concerning the hygienic care of intact infants found that of the 15 mothers who had intact sons, eight were not given any advice and the other seven were told to retract the foreskin during daily bathing. Of the 90 pediatricians surveyed, 47% wrongly believed that the foreskin should be easily retractable by 6 months, and a further 20% believed that it should be easily retractable by 1 year of age. This study had a small sample size, was conducted decades ago, and was limited to a region in the US with high circumcision rates. How relevant its results are today is unknown, and further studies should be conducted to determine the extent doctors and other health professionals are misinforming parents. Anecdotally at least, many parents in the US are misinformed by health care professionals regarding the proper care of the intact penis. See: Osborn, Metcalf and Mariani 1981.
31 Doctors Opposing Circumcision 2016.
32 Geisheker 2011.
33 Halata and Munger 1986.
34 Shih, Cold, and Yang 2013.
35 Ibid., 1786-1787.
36 Kelly et al., 2005.
37 Halata and Munger 1986.
38 von Frey 1894.
39 Halata and Munger 1986; Munger and Ide 1988.
40 Garcia-Mesa et al., 2021.
41 Bronselaer et al., 2013; Kim and Pang 2007; Fink, Carson, and DeVellis 2002.
42 Collins et al., 2002; Kigozi et al., 2008; Krieger et al., 2008.

43 Bronselaer et al., 2013, 7; Risser et al., 2004.
44 Sorrells et al., 2007.
45 Ibid.
46 Ibid., 868.
47 Bleustein et al., 2003; Payne et al., 2007.
48 Bleustein et al., 2005; Bossio, Pukall, and Steele 2016.
49 Bossio, Pukall, and Steele 2016.
50 Earp 2016a.
51 Kigozi et al., 2008.
52 Krieger et al., 2008.
53 American Academy of Pediatrics Task Force on Circumcision 2012.
54 Van Howe 2015.
55 Boyle 2015.
56 Frisch 2012.
57 Ibid.
58 I said Krieger et al (2013) appeared to imply circumcision resulted in condom use being easier over time because they did not state so outright. Rather they simply reported circumcised men found condoms easier to use when surveyed at 6, 12, 18 and 24 months, providing no further explanation, and leaving the reader to speculate as to why.
59 Bailey et al., 2007, 652.
60 Senkul et al., 2004.
61 Chung et al., 2015; Waldinger 2002.
62 Also called the bulbospongiosus muscle, the bulbocavernosus muscle is a muscle of the perineum, which is the area between the anus and the genitals. In males, it surrounds the bulb, which is the base of the penis located beneath the prostate.
63 Dean and Lue 2005.
64 Bird and Hanno 1998.
65 Sheu, Revenig, and Hsiao 2014, 13–29.
66 Podnar 2012.
67 Alp et al., 2014; Gao et al., 2015.
68 Frisch, Lindholm, and Grønbæk 2011.
69 O'Hara and O'Hara 1999; Tang and Khoo 2011.
70 Janssen et al., 2009; Jern et al., 2007.
71 Zhou et al., 2010.
72 Xin et al., 1996.
73 Paick, Jeong, and Park 1998; Rowland et al., 1993.
74 Goyal 2011.
75 Alp et al., 2014; Anaissie, Yafi, and Hellstrom 2016.
76 Gallo 2013.
77 Rowland et al., 1993, 196.

3. Cutting to cure?

1 American Academy of Pediatrics Task Force on Circumcision 1999.
2 American Academy of Pediatrics Task Force on Circumcision 2012.
3 Frisch et al., 2013.
4 Earp 2015b; Van Howe 2015.

5 Centers for Disease Control 2014, 4.
6 Svoboda and Van Howe 2014.
7 Langton 2015.
8 Svoboda and Van Howe 2014.
9 Darby 2003.
10 Darby 2005, 7; Dunsmuir and Gordon 1999.
11 Darby 2005, 7, 14–15.
12 Kellogg 1888, 295.
13 Bristow 1977, 28.
14 Maines 1999, 9–10.
15 Rodriguez 2008.
16 Rathmann 1959.
17 Little and White 2005.
18 Cathcart et al., 2003.
19 Piero and Alei 2008.
20 Agarwal, Mohta, and Anand 2005; Griffiths and Frank 1992; Huntley et al., 2003; Rickwood and Walker 1989.
21 Gonzalez and Ludwikowski 2010, 135; Porche 2006.
22 Zampieri et al., 2005. Although this study found topical steroids and stretching techniques are preferable to surgical correction, the average age of boys in the study was 7.6 years, suggesting the authors were not aware that it is common for the foreskin to remain fused to the glans until and well into puberty, and that they had mistaken normal non-retractile foreskin for phimosis.
23 Ashfield et al., 2003; Orsola, Caffaratti, and Garat 2000; Yang et al., 2005.
24 Munro et al., 2008.
25 Ying and Xiu-hua 1991. The balloon dilation was performed on boys aged 5 months to 12 years old, indicating the authors mistook normal non-retractile foreskin for phimosis. However, the technique remains a possible treatment option for young adult men who actually have phimosis, and studies should be performed to validate this treatment method.
26 Berdeu et al., 2001; Van Howe 1998.
27 Lichen sclerosus of the male genitalia is sometimes also referred to as balanitis xerotica obliterans.
28 Bunker and Shim 2015.
29 Fistarol and Itin 2013.
30 Ibid., 34–35.
31 Goldstein and Burrows 2007; Powell and Wojnarowska 1999.
32 Powell and Wojnarowska 1999.
33 Ibid., 38.
34 Kroft and Shier 2012; Windahl 2006.
35 For information on topical calcineurin inhibitors to treat genital lichen sclerosus see: Andreassi and Bilenchi 2013; Böhm, Frieling, and Luger 2003. Some have voiced concerns over the use of topical calcineurin inhibitors, which are known to have neoplastic potential, to treat lichen sclerosus, a dermatosis known to be precancerous. See: Bunker 2011. This concern is valid, although it remains unclear how the risk of malignancy resulting from the use of topical calcineurin inhibitors compares to the risk of malignancy resulting from

chronic inflammation. If steroids fail to control inflammation it may be that calcineurin inhibitors are the next best option if they can reduce the overall risk of malignancy. Ultimately, it is for the patient to decide if they prefer the risk of penile cancer developing to the risks of circumcision. In any case, topical steroids should remain the first line of treatment.

36 Catterall and Oates 1962.
37 Neill et al., 2010, 674.
38 Helm 1991.
39 Lipscombe et al., 1997.
40 Meeuwis et al., 2011; Shim et al., 2016.
41 Porter and Bunker 2001.
42 Hoshi, Usui, and Terachi 2008; Leal-Khouri and Hruza 1994; Neill et al., 2010.
43 Balato et al., 2009.
44 Tobian and Gray 2011.
45 Castellsagué et al., 2002.
46 Senkomago et al., 2015; Weaver et al., 2004.
47 Van Howe 2007.
48 Harper et al., 2004; Koutsky et al., 2002; Villa et al., 2005.
49 Brotherton et al., 2011.
50 Larke et al., 2011; Schoen et al., 2000.
51 US population 321,418,820 (source: World Bank) / 2 x sex ratio .97 (source: Central Intelligence Agency: The World Factbook) = 165,679,804 men / 2080 new cases p/y (See: American Cancer Society) = 1 case per 79,654 men.
52 AU population in 2009: 21,691,700 (source: World Bank) / 2 x sex ratio 1 (source: Central Intelligence Agency: The World Factbook) = 10,845,850 men / 82 new cases in 2009 (See: Australian Institute of Health and Welfare and Australasian Association of Cancer Registries) = 1 case per 132,266 men.
53 UK population in 2014: 64,613,160 (source: World Bank) / 2 x sex ratio .99 (source: Central Intelligence Agency: The World Factbook) = 32,632,909 men / 550 new cases p/y (National Health Service Inform 2020) = 1 case per 59,332 men; Dave et al., 2003.
54 Dave et al., 2003; Morris et al., 2016; Richters et al., 2006; Spilsbury et al., 2003.
55 Larke et al., 2011.
56 Castellsagué et al., 2002.
57 Ornellas and Ornellas 2018.
58 Voris, Visintin, and Reis 2018.
59 American Cancer Society 2020a.
60 American Cancer Society 2020b.
61 American Cancer Society 2020c.
62 American Academy of Pediatrics Task Force on Circumcision 2012.
63 Learman 1999.
64 Royal Australasian College of Physicians 2010.
65 Shingleton and Heath Jr 1996.
66 Ibid.
67 Misra, Chaturvedi, and Misra 2004.
68 Van Howe and Hodges 2006.
69 Morris and Wiswell 2013.

70   Harper and Fowlis 2007.

71   Robinson et al., 2014.

72   Despite evidence indicating that urine might not be sterile as the prevailing medical wisdom suggests, and that we have been culturing urine under the wrong conditions to get the normal flora in it to grow, under the culture conditions normally used urine doesn't grow anything unless it is 'bad bacteria'. However, the bacteria under the foreskin can contaminate the urine sample and grow when cultured, which can make it appear as though there is an infection in the urinary tract, because no growth is expected in 'sterile' urine samples.

73   Cold 2001; Van Howe 2005.

74   Chessare 1992.

75   Bartman 2001; Canfield 2001.

76   Harper and Fowlis 2007; Robinson et al., 2014.

77   Kwak et al., 2004.

78   Mishra and Motiwala 2010, 307–311.

79   Ibid., 309.

80   Carmack, Notini, and Earp 2015.

81   Örtqvist et al., 2016.

82   Gray and Boston 2003.

83   Shenoy et al., 2015.

84   Dockray, Finlayson, and Gordon 2011; Rajan, McNeill, and Turner 2006.

85   Frisch and Simonsen 2021.

86   Ibid.

87   Cook, Koutsky, and Holmes 1994; Dickson et al., 2008; Tobian et al., 2009; Van Howe 1999; Weiss et al., 2006.

88   Iwasaki 2010.

89   Fink 1986.

90   Baggaley, White, and Boily 2010; Iwasaki 2010; Karim and Gita 1998.

91   Doerner et al., 2013; Gust et al., 2010; Jameson et al., 2010; Millett et al., 2007; Sanchez et al., 2011.

92   Drain et al., 2006; Halperin and Bailey 1999.

93   Auvert et al., 2005.

94   Bailey et al., 2007.

95   Gray et al., 2007.

96   Van Howe 2011.

97   Ibid.

98   Biryabarema 2012.

99   The Pew Global Attitudes Project 2007, 35–36.

100 Ramjee and Gouws 2002.

101 Brody and Potterat 2003.

102 Although this too would have been limited to cases of assumed insertive anal sex, as receptive anal sex indicates someone else with a penis was involved.

103 In fairness, it has been argued that the failure to control for men who have sex with men is not the problem some make it out to be, because randomization of trial participants would evenly distribute sexual behavior between groups (Wamai et al., 2012, 106). Counter to this argument is that "it would still be a problem for making generalizations based on sample characteristics, because if you don't

know who was in your sample along a theoretically relevant dimension then you can't extrapolate along that dimension." Brian Earp, Associate Director Yale-Hastings Program in Ethics and Health Policy, Email to author October 2, 2020.

104 It could be (and indeed has been) argued these drop outs were not statistically significant between groups, with 9.5%, 9.2% and 8.2% of the intact control groups, and 6.5%, 9.0% and 9.1% of the circumcised intervention groups dropping out, for the South African, Ugandan and Kenyan RCTs respectively. See: Wamai et al., 2012 102, 123. However, such an argument misses the point entirely, because the number of dropouts needn't have been statistically significant *between groups* to have a significant impact on the validity of the overall results. Here's why: in the South African, Ugandan, and Kenyan trials, 49 (2.9%), 45 (1.8%) and 47 (3.4%) of men in the intact control groups, and 20 (1.2%), 22 (0.89%) and 22 (1.6%) of men in the circumcised intervention groups acquired HIV. This represents an absolute difference in HIV acquisition of just 0.7%, 0.91% and 1.8% between the control and intervention groups for the South African, Ugandan, and Kenyan RCTs, respectively. Meaning that the rate of dropouts was several times greater than the supposed "protective effect" seen.

105 Boyle and Hill 2011, 322.

106 Auvert et al., 2005, 1120.

107 Ibid.

108 10 - 5 = 5 fewer relapses per 100 people = 5% reduction.

109 5 / 10 = .5 x 100 = 50% reduction compared to first treatment regimen.

110 ((137/5,497) - (64/5,411)) x 100 = 1.31%.

111 Nayan et al., 2021.

112 UNAIDS 2011.

113 Wawer et al., 2009.

114 Ibid., 235.

115 Kojima and Klausner 2016; Lal et al., 2017; McCormack et al., 2016.

116 Bavinton et al., 2018; Rodger et al., 2016.

117 Dube 2014.

118 George et al., 2016.

119 Darby 2014.

120 Fish et al., 2020.

4. A bloody mess

1 Studies testing the effect of glucose and sucrose on pain relief have suffered from small sample sizes, and from methodologies with the systematic error of assuming that a reduction in crying time or other behavioral changes are adequate markers of pain relief. The evidence indicates otherwise.

We know that although pain generally evokes cortical and behavioral changes, that pain can be processed at the cortical level without producing behavioral changes. Indeed, cortical pain responses have been recorded in infants who did not display a change in facial expression (Slater et al., 2008). This indicates what needs to be considered is where sugars like glucose and sucrose act in the brain. A study of infants that looked at the effect of sucrose on pain relief by measuring brain activity found no significant difference in nociceptive brain activity after noxious heel lance between the sucrose and control group (Slater et al., 2010).

In rats given oral sucrose it has been shown that decreased nociceptive behavior persists after midbrain transection, which suggests the forebrain is not needed for this effect (Anseloni et al., 2005). Therefore, sucrose could inhibit facial motor activity by mediating brainstem inhibition of behavior, despite strong pain activation occurring in the forebrain.

This means it's possible for infants on sugar to feel pain even though they can't express it, which is just the sort of thing you'd miss if the focus of your study were crying time or heart rate instead of pain activation in the brain.

2   Ryan and Finer 1994; Wellington and Rieder 1993.
3   Serour et al., 1998.
4   Holman, Lewis, and Ringler 1995.
5   Wan 2002.
6   Weiss 1962, 36.
7   Okeke, Asinobi, and Ikuerowo 2006.
8   Kulkarni and Lusher 2001.
9   Food and Drug Administration 2009.
10 Rodriguez et al., 2010.
11 Ibid.
12 Kearney, Sharathkumar, and Rodriguez 2015.
13 Isaacs et al., 2003.
14 Ibid.
15 Some have acknowledged circumcision increases the risk of MRSA infection, but nonetheless argued (as one might expect from American doctors) for better infection control practices rather than forgoing circumcision (Nguyen et al., 2007; Pelton 2009). This is unfortunate, because while it is true the disuse of multiple-dose lidocaine vials and improved hygiene practices will reduce the risk of infection, there remain many opportunities for infection to occur, and the risk of infection is best reduced by not performing unnecessary invasive surgical procedures in the first place.
16 Consolini 2013.
17 Corbett and Humphrey 2003.
18 Baba et al., 2002; Carey and Long 2010; Chambers, 2005.
19 Bliss, Healey, and Waldhausen 1997.
20 Gemmel and Boyle 2000, 241–252.
21 Demirdover et al., 2013; Xie, Li, and Li 2013.
22 Yildirim, Akoz, and Akan 2000.
23 Kon 1983.
24 Eroğlu et al., 2009.
25 Alter, Horton, and Horton 1994; Sivakumar, Brown, and Kangesu 2004.
26 Ponsky et al., 2000; Snodgrass 2006.
27 Kaplan 1983.
28 Lackey, Mannion, and Kerr 1968; Sancaktutar et al., 2011.
29 The pathophysiology of meatal stenosis is debatable. It may result from meatitis or ischaemia of the meatal mucosa following damage to the frenular artery. Whatever the case, the rarity of meatal stenosis in those who are intact, compared to its high frequency in those who are not, suggests in most cases the causative factor is related to circumcision.

30 Persad et al., 1995.
31 Van Howe 2006.
32 Mihssin, Moorthy, and Houghton 1999.
33 Dwyer et al., 2016; Jee and Millar 1990.
34 Eason, McDonnell, and Clark 1994.
35 RT. "Swiss court acquits doctor who cut off 4yo's penis in botched circumcision," RT.com, April 19, 2007. https://www.rt.com/news/385325-doctor-circumcision-switzerland-ruling
36 News.com.au 2016; Associated Press 2014; Davies 2015; Nagesh 2016.
37 Krill, Palmer, and Palmer 2011.
38 It is surprisingly difficult to find any examples in the medical literature, but curvature of the penis following circumcision is a well-known complication among urologists (Collins 2014; Kaplan 1983).
39 Cilento, Holmes, and Canning 1999.
40 Altokhais, T.I. 2017.
41 Arda et al., 2000; Couper, R.T.L. 2000.
42 Odemis, Sommez, and Aslan 2004.
43 Bollinger 2010.
44 Taddio et al., 1997.
45 Boyle 2003.
46 Boyle et al., 2002; Ramos and Boyle 2000.
47 Abdel-Azim 2012; Haseena 1999; Lever et al., 2018; Merritt 2011; Mulongo, Martin, and McAndrew 2014.
48 Glover 1929.
49 Goldman 1999. For those wanting to learn more about the psychological consequences of circumcision, I recommend reading Goldman 1997.
50 Carlisle 2016.
51 Greer, Mohl, and Sheley 1982.

5. A view to a cut

1 Dover 1989, 125.
2 Ibid., 125, 127.
3 Oredsson 2015.
4 Ibid.
5 Money 1991.
6 Harryman 2004.
7 Lauder 2016.
8 Maeda, Chari, and Elixhauser 2012; Merrill, Nagamine, and Steiner 2008.
9 The American Society of Plastic Surgeons doesn't publish cosmetic genital procedures in its annual plastic surgery statistical reports. Thankfully the American Society for Aesthetic Plastic Surgery also publishes annual statistical reports, which have included data on labiaplasty since 2013. Their reports indicate there were 10,774 labiaplasty procedures performed in the US in 2016, up from 8,745 in 2015, 7,535 in 2014, and 5,070 in 2013 (American Society for Aesthetic Plastic Surgery 2016).
10 This may or may not be true, depending on how many cases of backyard female genital mutilation go unreported. As with all unreported problems it is impossible

to know their scale, but it is possible in some regions they outnumber cosmetic procedures. Of course, in the parts of the world where female genital cutting is common, it is almost always involuntary.

11　Feder 1995.

12　American Society of Plastic and Reconstructive Surgeons 1982, 4–5. For an analysis of the FDA's response see: Jacobson 2000.

13　Cohen 1994, 169; See also: Weisman 1993.

14　The Guardian 2011.

15　IBISWorld 2019.

16　American Society of Plastic Surgeons 2019.

17　American Society of Plastic Surgeons 2018.

18　Silvestre et al., 2014.

19　Circumcision Center, 993-C Johnson Ferry Rd NE, Suite 225, Atlanta, Georgia. https://www.circumcisioncenter.com

20　Gentle Circumcision, 9808 Venice Blvd., Suite 602, Culver City, California. https://www.gentlecircumcision.com

21　Campo-Flores 2014.

22　Queensland Circumcision Service, C3 528 Compton Road, Sunnybank Hills, Queensland. https://www.circumcisionsqld.com.au

23　Figuratively speaking, of course.

24　Nahm, Zhou, and Falanga 2002.

25　Zenbio. Human dermal fibroblasts. Cryopreserved, neonatal dermal fibroblasts. Item# DFN-F http://www.zen-bio.com/products/cells/fibroblasts.php; ScienCell. Human dermal fibroblasts – neonatal. Catalog# 2310 http://www.sciencellonline.com/products-services/stem-cells/human-dermal-fibroblasts-neonatal.html; ThermoFisher. Human dermal fibroblasts, neonatal (HDFn). Catalog# C0045C. https://www.thermofisher.com/order/catalog/product/C0045C

26　Valveta®, also known as ICX-RHY, Ember Therapeutics acquired Vavelta® from Intercytex in 2016 (Ember Therapeutics 2016). For product cost, see: Consulting Room: The Cosmetic Guru. Vavelta®: Product Summary. Consultingroom.com Ltd. http://www.consultingroom.com/Treatment/Vavelta

27　Hovatta et al., 2003.

28　Knight 1976.

29　Harding, Sumner, and Cardinal 2013.

30　Euringer 2006.

31　Naughton, Mansbridge, and Gentzkow 1997.

6. Copy cuts

1　Jackson 1997, 119–121.

2　Bisono et al., 2012.

3　Tiemstra 1999.

4　Williamson and Paul 1988.

5　Ibid.

6　Ibid.

7　Davies 1996, 543.

8　Brown and Brown 1987; Chantry et al., 2010; See also numbers from a Roy Morgan Poll as reported in an episode of the Channel 10 television show *Can of*

Worms, which aired in 2012. https://vimeo.com/channels/419158/53302461

9 Davis 2013.

10 Ibid.

11 Alexander, Storm, and Cooper 2014.

12 Studies involving self-reporting can be unreliable because they are subjective (i.e. what one individual considers 'teasing' another considers joking). Alexander, Storm, and Cooper (2014) provided a definition of teasing to account for this. However, another aspect of the study that could affect reliability is that the researchers were requiring people to remember things that happened years ago. It's human nature that our memories are terrible at the best of times, but this is especially true when having to remember events that occurred a long time ago. One is left wondering why they didn't simply ask a cohort of high school students to report their more recent locker room experiences.

13 Another place one might expect such locker room teasing over circumcision status is Israel. A Jewish friend who served in the Israeli army informed me, "They'll laugh at him when he's in the army" is a surprisingly common argument in Israeli circumcision debates. My friend once held what he calls "a highly informal survey on this matter", and the number of reported instances of people laughing at others' penises in showers – or indeed acknowledging in any way whatsoever the existence of said penises – was zero. The common attitude seemed to be "why would I look at another guy's penis?"

14 World Health Organization 2007.

15 Royal Australasian College of Physicians 2010.

16 Bartholomew et al., 2011, 222–225.

17 Darby 2011.

18 Bartholomew et al., 2011, 222.

19 Center for Disease Control and Prevention 2010.

20 Maeda, Chari, and Elixhauser 2012, 1–13.

21 Ku et al., 2003.

22 Kim, Koo, and Pang 2012; Pang and Kim 2002.

23 Darby and Cozijn 2013.

24 Ibid., 8.

25 Ibid., 2–3, 8.

26 Douglas 1996.

27 Gollaher 1994, 23.

28 Gollaher 1994.

7. On religious freedom, rights, and the law

1 Paterson 2012.

2 Swatek-Evenstein 2013, 46.

3 Ibid., 46.

4 Bundesgesetzblatt 2012.

5 Merkel and Putzke 2013.

6 Hartmann 2013.

7 Freeman 2002, 102; Universal Declaration of Human Rights (1948). (GA Res 217 A III) Article 1.

8 Vienna Declaration and Programme of Action: adopted by the World Conference on Human Rights in Vienna on 25 June 1993.

9 'Covenant' is synonymous with 'Convention'. Conventions carry more weight than Declarations because they are legally binding to governments that have ratified them.

10 World Health Organization 2008, 8–10.

11 Svoboda, Adler, and Van Howe 2013.

12 International Covenant on Civil and Political Rights, Article 18(4); 1952 Protocol of the European Convention on Human Rights, Article 2.

13 Convention on the Rights of the Child, Nov. 20 1989, 1577 UNTS 3, art 14(3); International Covenant on Civil and Political Rights, art 18(1-3).

14 Convention on the Rights of the Child, art 19(1).

15 International Covenant on Civil and Political Rights, art 9; European Convention for the Protection of Human Rights and Fundamental Freedoms, Nov. 4 1950, 213 UNTS 221, art 5.

16 International Covenant on Civil and Political Rights, art 7; European Convention for the Protection of Human Rights and Fundamental Freedoms, art 3; Convention on the Rights of the Child, art 37(a).

17 International Covenant on Economic, Social and Cultural Rights, Dec. 12 1966, 993 UNTS 3, art 12; Convention on the Rights of the Child, art 24(1).

18 International Covenant on Civil and Political Rights, art 18(1); European Convention for the Protection of Human Rights and Fundamental Freedoms art 9; Convention on the Rights of the Child, art 14(1).

19 Convention on the Rights of the Child, art 19(1).

20 United Nations (Committee on the Rights of the Child) 2011, para 17.

21 United Nations (Human Rights Committee) 2014, para 9.

22 Convention on the Rights of the Child, art 18(1).

23 United Nations (Committee on the Rights of the Child) 2007, para 18; United Nations (Committee on the Rights of the Child) 2011, para 23.

24 United Nations (Commission on Human Rights) 2005, para 39.

25 United Nations (Human Rights Committee) 2000, para 11; United Nations (Human Rights Council) 2010, para 201.

26 United Nations (Human Rights Council) 2016, para 48; See also: United Nations (Human Rights Council) 2013a, paras 77 and 88.

27 United Nations (Human Rights Council) 2008, para 53.

28 United Nations (General Assembly) 2011, para 9.

29 Convention on the Rights of the Child, art 24(3).

30 International Covenant on Economic, Social, and Cultural Rights (n 57) art 12(a); Convention on the Rights of the Child (n 7) art 24.

31 Bollinger 2010.

32 United Nations (General Assembly) 2003, paras 1 and 2.

33 Fox and Thomson 2012.

34 United Nations (Human Rights Council) 2013b, para 43.

35 Swatek-Evenstein 2013.

36 When parents label their children as being a Jewish child, a Muslim child, or a child of any other religion, they are making a conceptual error. There's no such thing as religious children because children are too young to understand religious concepts, just as Marxist or utilitarian children don't exist, because they're too young to understand concepts of political and moral philosophy. There are no

religious children, only children of religious parents. Of course children being too young to understand religious concepts doesn't stop people from labeling them as religious anyway. If a child is mature enough to engage in an intelligible conversation about a subject like religion or politics, it seems fair to argue they are capable of identifying with a particular religious or political group. I suspect this excludes pre-pubescent children, and probably in most cases it also excludes adolescents.

37 *Gender Identity, Gender Expression and Sex Characteristic Act 2015* (Malta).

38 Queensland Law Reform Commission 1993, 3–16.

39 Marshall 2012.

40 Parliamentary Assembly, Council of Europe. Assembly debate on 1 October 2013 (31st Sitting) (see Doc. 13297, report of the Committee on Social Affairs, Health and Sustainable Development, rapporteur: Ms Rupprecht). Text adopted by the Assembly on 1 October 2013 (31st Sitting). See also Recommendation 2023 (2013). http://assembly.coe.int/nw/xml/XRef/Xref-XML2HTML-en.asp?fileid=20174&lang=en

41 Lindboe et al., 2013.

42 OLG Frankfurt A.M., Beschluss vom 21. 8. 2007, Az. 4 W 12/07.

43 OLG Hamm, Beschluss vom 30. 8. 2013, Az. 3 UF 133/13.

44 [UK] Royal Courts of Justice, In the matter of B and G (Children) (No 2), Neutral Citation Number (2015) EWFC 3, Case Number LJ13C00295, para 69.

45 [UK] High Court of Justice, Family Division, Re L and B (Children), Neutral Citation Number (2016) EWHC 849 (Fam), April 5, 2016.

46 *Children's Act No. 38 of 2005* (South Africa), ss12(8-10). See also: *General Regulations Regarding Children 2010* (South Africa), Chapter 1, Part II.

47 18 USC Sec. 116, Female genital mutilation, Congressional Findings, Section (3).

48 Svoboda, Adler, and Van Howe 2013.

49 Bond 1999.

50 *United States of America v. Nagarwala, et al.*, Criminal No. 17-CR-20274 (E.D. Mich., 2018).

51 Brigman 1985.

52 California Penal Code Section 273.4

53 California Penal Code Section 273a(b) (child abuse); California Penal Code Section 240 (assault); California Penal Code Section §§ 11165.1, 1165,1(a),(b) (3); Svoboda, Adler, and Van Howe 2013, 273.

54 Svoboda, Adler, and Van Howe, 2013, 273.

55 Idaho Criminal Code § 18-1506A(2)(b).

56 720 Illinois Compiled Statutes §§ 5/12-32(b) and 5/12-33(b) (2).

57 Mississippi Code § 97-5-39(2)(b)(iv).

58 24 Delaware Code § 1703(10).

59 Minnesota Statutes § 147.09(10).

60 Montana Code § 37-3-103(1)(g).

61 Wisconsin Statutes § 448.03(2)(g).

62 McDonald 2010.

63 The Economist 2016.

64 60 Minutes Australia 2013.

65 Some people will no doubt pretend to want their sons circumcised for religious

reasons, but this barrier will likely serve as a sufficient deterrent for many, and one can imagine requiring rabbis and imams to sign forms confirming people's religious affiliation.

66   The definition of 'medical necessity' in relation to medical interventions must be over and above that which is merely 'therapeutic' (i.e., that which conveys some health benefits). The necessity of a medical intervention must be defined by it being *urgently* required and *non-deferrable*, such that the intervention cannot be delayed until a minor has the capacity to express a view or provide their own informed consent, due to the immediate or near immediate and grave health risks posed by such delay. All medical emergencies will involve medically necessary interventions, but it is possible to imagine medically necessary interventions that do not yet meet the threshold of a medical emergency, hence the need for a statutory definition of medical necessity to guide clinical practice in adhering to legislation outlawing non-consensual, medically unnecessary/deferrable alterations of sex characteristics.

8. A religious rite that's wrong

1   Zwi Werblowsky and Wigoder 1997, 161.
2   Elseesy 2014.
3   Grisaru, Lezer, and Belmaker 1997.
4   Genesis 17:5, World English Bible.
5   Ibid., 15–16, World English Bible.
6   Ibid., 4, World English Bible. 'Father of multitudes' also happens to be the meaning of Abram's new name, Abraham.
7   Ibid., 10–11, World English Bible.
8   Ibid., 12–14, World English Bible.
9   Ibid., 12, World English Bible.
10 Glick 2005, 15.
11 Mack 1915, 18.
12 Newman 2016.
13 Exodus 4:24, World English Bible.
14 Ibid., 25–26, World English Bible.
15 Joshua 5:2, World English Bible.
16 Finklestein and Silberman 2001.
17 The argument from tradition is a logical fallacy discussed in Chapter 6.
18 Glick 2005, 44.
19 HSV-1 is the virus that causes cold sores, and is of little concern when infection occurs in adults. HSV-1 is not to be confused with HSV-2, which is the type that causes genital herpes, and can cause a potentially fatal infection in newborns if they pass through the birth canal of an infected mother. If you have genital herpes and are pregnant or planning to get pregnant, see your doctor.
20 Blank et al., 2012; James 2012; Rubin and Lanzkowsky 2000.
21 Babylonian Talmud, Sabbath 133b.
22 The New York Times Editorial Board 2015.
23 Ibid.
24 Levenson 1993, 50–52.
25 Leviticus 19:23–25, World English Bible.
26 Glick 2005, 18.

27 Leviticus 12:1–5, World English Bible.
28 Rabbi Dovid Gutnick, East Melbourne Synagogue, Emails to the author, September 24 and 26, 2016.
29 Maimonides, Moses 1904, 504.
30 Ibid., 503.
31 Ibid.
32 Ibid.
33 Ibid.
34 CTForum 2009.
35 Jewish Business News 2016; Ahituv 2012.
36 You can watch Lisa Braver Moss' presentation to the 13th International Symposium on Genital Autonomy and Children's Rights on YouTube: https://www.youtube.com/watch?v=8q9qmp0qjng&list= PLmrnvFzPoElqHDRiboV5R9 PPsogSp_k_v&index=3
37 Acts 10:1–8, World English Bible.
38 Ibid., 9–15, World English Bible.
39 Ibid., 17–23, World English Bible.
40 Ibid., 47–48, World English Bible.
41 Acts 11:3, World English Bible.
42 Acts 15:6–21, World English Bible.
43 Ibid., 19–29, World English Bible.
44 Titus 1:10–11, World English Bible.
45 Philippians 3:2, World English Bible. Some versions refer to "mutilation" instead of false circumcision".
46 Matthew 15:26, World English Bible.
47 Eternal World Television Network.
48 May we also not forget the many homosexuals, disabled people, and those otherwise deemed undesirable who were also murdered in the Holocaust.
49 Pope Paul VI 1965.
50 The Catholic Leader 2002.
51 Pope Benedict XVI 2007.
52 A catechism is a religious instruction.
53 Bordwell 2006, 494.
54 You can hear the haunting sound of the last Vatican castrato Alessandro Moreschi, the only castrato whose voice was ever recorded, on YouTube: https://www.youtube.com/watch?t=19&v=slhhg8sI6Ds
55 Aldeeb Abu-Sahlieh 2012, 136–140.
56 Ibid., 140–143.
57 World Health Organization 2007.
58 In some places *khitan* is used to refer both to male and female circumcision.
59 Rizvi et al., 1999.
60 Dirie and Lindmark 1991.
61 Ibid.
62 Lightfoot-Klein 1991.
63 Sahih Muslim 257b, Book 2, Hadith 65.
64 Sahih al-Bukhari 5890, Book 77, Hadith 107; Sahih Muslim 261a, Book 2, Hadith 71.

65 Sunan Abi Dawud 5271, Book 43, Hadith 499.
66 For an analysis of why this hadith lacks authenticity see: Lutfi al-Sabbagh 1996, 17–23.
67 El-Damanhoury 2013.
68 Office of the Senior Coordinator for International Women's Issues 2001.
69 Alsibiana and Rouzi 2010.
70 Dehghankhalili et al., 2015.
71 WADI 2010.
72 Rashid, Patil, and Valimalar 2010.
73 Office of the Senior Coordinator for International Women's Issues 2001.
74 Merli 2008.
75 Marranci 2014.
76 Gibeau 1998.
77 Dasgupta 2011.

9. Not so clear cut

1 Infant ankle bands can be purchased at TLCTugger.com.
2 Los Angeles County Superior Court. No. SOC 36797, September 1979, 17 Verdict Report 24 (April 8, 1980), The Exchange cases.
3 Llewellyn 1995.
4 Reinert 2001.
5 Georganne Chapin, Founding Executive Director of Intact America, Email to author, November 18, 2016.
6 Ibid.
7 Ibid.
8 British Medical Association 2004.
9 Mill 1859.
10 Lyons 2013.
11 Mandela 1994, 30–36.
12 Ibid.
13 Ibid.
14 Ibid.
15 Ibid.
16 Ibid.
17 Greer 2007, 119–134.
18 Ibid., 121.
19 Ibid., 126.
20 Some readers will be correcting me. The other half of the glass isn't empty because there are air molecules in it. I am using some creative license okay, just roll with it.
21 Wong 1993, 39.
22 Even if it did follow that just because people hold to different truths that there exists no objective truth of the matter, it still couldn't entail tolerance without contradiction, for one cannot argue that no non-relative moral principles exist, only then to argue that we must always tolerate other cultures, which is itself a non-relative claim (Williams 1976, 34–35).
23 Midgley 1993, 176.

24 Hume 1739, 335.

25 Earp 2016b; Harris 2010.

26 This of course is where many philosophers would point out that Hume's is-ought problem applies, because we first need to make the value judgment that we ought to value the wellbeing of conscious creatures, so all subsequent "oughts" – such as since we value wellbeing then we ought not to mutilate children – can only be reached through this previous value judgment that is itself not based on fact. Stated another way by the philosopher Tibor Machan, the is-ought problem "expresses the philosophical claim that a conclusion that contains moral terms such as "ought to" or "ought not to" cannot be *deduced* from premises that lack those moral terms, because a valid deductive argument can only have in its conclusion components that are fully supported by its premises" (Machan 2008, 105). Let's unpack that a bit because Machan used a lot of philosophical language. An *argument* attempts to convince its reader or listener of a claim by providing reasons for believing it. Arguments consist of premises and a conclusion. The premises of an argument are the reasons or evidence that lead to a conclusion. A *valid* argument is one in which it is impossible for the premises to be true but the conclusion false. An *invalid* argument is one in which it is still possible for the conclusion to be false even if all the premises are true. And a *deductive* argument is one in which the certainty of the conclusion is guaranteed by the certainty of its premises. If you've ever read or watched Sherlock Holmes, you will know of Holmes' many 'deductions', but what Holmes is engaging in most of the time is *inductive* arguments, which is when the truth of an argument's premises makes its conclusion likely or probable but does not guarantee it.

Hume's is-ought problem simply points out that it is impossible to make deductive moral conclusions when the premises are non-moral (or factual). But this does not mean that such moral arguments cannot be valid. As for the problem faced by all goal-dependent oughts, namely why we should value the goal in the first place, I have no doubt this is a question that can only be answered by philosophy, and I accept this value judgment about goals first needing to be made.

10. Toward the final cut

1 The term 'intactivist' was coined in 1995 by a New Yorker called Richard DeSeabra. Marilyn Milos, Founding Executive Director of NOCIRC, Email to author, April 1, 2017.

2 I had the pleasure of meeting Marilyn when I spoke at the 13th International Symposium on Genital Autonomy and Children's Rights held at Boulder University, Colorado, in 2014.

3 15 Square is a reference to the upper limit of square inches of foreskin tissue lost by circumcision.

4 Hemmelgarn 2016.

5 Roberts 2021.

Bibliography

60 Minutes Australia, Interview by Tara Brown. 2013. "The case against circumcision: Barrister Paul Mason." *YouTube*, March 3, 2013. https://www.youtube.com/watch?v=Uc1L0lVVDS8

Abdel-Azim, Said. 2012. Psychosocial and sexual aspects of female circumcision. *African Journal of Urology* 19 (3): 141–142.

Agarwal, A., A. Mohta, and R. Anand. 2005. Preputial retraction in children. *Journal of Indian Association of Pediatric Surgeons, Expanded Academic ASAP* 10 (2): 89–91.

AHA Foundation. "FGM legislation by state." https://www.theahafoundation.org/female-genital-mutilation/fgm-legislation-by-state

Ahituv, Netta. 2012. "Even in Israel, more and more parents choose not to circumcise their sons." *Haaretz*, June 14, 2012. http://www.haaretz.com/israel-news/even-in-israel-more-and-more-parents-choose-not-to-circumcise-their-sons-1.436421

Aldeeb Abu-Sahlieh, Sami. 2012. *Male and female circumcision: religious, medical, social and legal debate* (Second edition). Centre of Arab and Islamic Law 136–140.

Alexander, S.E., D.W. Storm, and C.S. Cooper. 2014. Teasing in school locker rooms regarding penile appearance. *The Journal of Urology* 193: 983–988.

Alibhai, Shabbir M.H. 1995. Female circumcision not in Qur'an. *Canadian Medical Association Journal* 152 (8): 1190.

Alp, B.F., S. Uguz, E. Malkoc, F. Ates, F. Dursun, S. Okcelik, H. Kocoglu, and A.K. Karademir. 2014. Does circumcision have a relationship with ejaculation time? Premature ejaculation evaluated using new diagnostic tools. *International Journal of Impotence Research* 26: 121–123.

Alsibiana, S.A., and A.A. Rouzi. 2010. Sexual function in women with female genital mutilation. *Fertility and Sterility* 93 (3): 722–724.

Alter, G.J., C.E. Horton, and C.E. Jr. Horton. 1994. Buried penis as a contraindication for circumcision. *Journal of the American College of Surgeons* 178 (5): 487–490.

Altokhais, T.I. 2017. Electrosurgery use in circumcision in children: is it safe? *Urology Annals* 9 (1): 1–3.

Aly, Waleed. 2013. "Why we should stop using the phrase 'female genital mutilation'." *RN Drive*, April 15, 2013. http://www.abc.net.au/radionational/programs/drive/female-circumcision-debate/4630478

American Academy of Pediatrics Committee on Bioethics. 2010. Policy statement – ritual genital cutting of female minors. *Pediatrics* 125: 1088–1093.

American Academy of Pediatrics Task Force on Circumcision. 1999. Circumcision policy statement. *Pediatrics* 103 (3): 686–693.

——. 2012. Technical report: Male circumcision. *Pediatrics* 130: e756–785.

American Cancer Society. (Last reviewed 2018, June 25, estimate for 2018). What are the key statistics about penile cancer? http://www.cancer.org/cancer/penilecancer/detailedguide/penile-cancer-key-statistics

——. 2020a. What are the key statistics about cervical cancer? (Last revised 2020, July 30) http://www.cancer.org/cancer/cervicalcancer/detailedguide/cervical-cancer-key-statistics

——. 2020b. What are the key statistics about breast cancer? (Last revised 2020, January 8) http://www.cancer.org/cancer/breastcancer/detailedguide/breast-cancer-key-statistics

——. 2020c. Penile cancer: What is penile cancer? (Last revised 2020, January 8) http://www.cancer.org/cancer/penilecancer/detailedguide/penile-cancer-key-statistics

American Society for Aesthetic Plastic Surgery. 2016. Cosmetic Surgery National Data Bank Statistics (2013, 2014, 2015 & 2016).

American Society of Plastic and Reconstructive Surgeons. 1982. Comments of the American Society of Plastic and Reconstructive Surgeons on the Proposed Classification of Inflatable Breast Prosthesis (Docket No. 78N-2653) and Silicone Gel-Filled Breast Prosthesis (Docket No. 78N-2654). 47, *Fed. Reg.* 2810, January 19, 1982, submitted to the FDA July 1, 1982 (unpublished document).

American Society of Plastic Surgeons. 2018. Plastic surgery statistics report: National clearinghouse of plastic surgery procedural statistics.

——. 2019. About APS: History of ASPS. (Last updated 2019). http://www.plasticsurgery.org/about-asps/history-of-asps.html?sub=ASPRS#content

Anaissie, J., F.A. Yafi, and W.J.G. Hellstrom. 2016. Surgery is not indicated for the treatment of premature ejaculation. *Translational Andrology and Urology* 5 (4): 607–612.

Andreassi, M. and R. Bilenchi. 2013. Topical pimecrolimus in the treatment of genital lichen sclerosus. *Expert Review in Dermatology* 8 (5): 443.

Anseloni, V.C.Z., K. Ren, R. Dubner, and M. Ennis. 2005. A brainstem substrate for analgesia elicited by intraoral sucrose. *Neuroscience* 133 (1): 231–243.

Arda, I.S., N. Özbek, E. Akpek, and E. Ersoy. 2000. Toxic neonatal methaemoglobinaemia after prilocaine administration for circumcision. *British Journal of Urology International* 85 (9): 1.

Ashfield, J.E., K.R. Nickel, D.R. Siemens, A.E. MacNeily, and J.C. Nickel. 2003. Treatment of phimosis with topical steroids in 194 children. *The Journal of Urology* 169: 1106–1108.

Associated Press. 2014. "Patient, 56, wakes up from routine circumcision to find his penis amputated." *Daily Mail*, July 25, 2014. http://www.dailymail.co.uk/news/article-2704558/Alabama-man-claims-penis-mistakenly-amputated.html

Associated Press in Boynton Beach, Florida. 2015. "Florida four-year-old at centre of circumcision battle." *The Guardian*, January 20, 2015. http://www.theguardian.com/us-news/2015/jan/19/circumcision-florida-four-year-old-battle

Australian Institute of Health and Welfare and Australasian Association of Cancer Registries 2012. *Cancer in Australia: an overview*, 2012. Cancer series no. 74. Cat. no. CAN 70. Canberra, AIHW.

Auvert, B., D. Taljaard, E. Lagarde, J. Sobngwi-Tambekou, R. Sitta, and A. Puren. 2005. Randomized, controlled intervention trial of male circumcision for reduction of HIV infection risk: ANRS 1265 trial. *PLoS Medicine* 2 (11): 1112–1122.

Baba, T., F. Takeuchi, M. Kuroda, H. Yuzawa, K. Aoki, A. Oguchi, Y. Nagai, et al. 2002. Genome and virulence determinants of high-virulence community acquired MRSA. *The Lancet* 359: 1919–1927.

Baggaley, R.F., R.G. White, and M.C. Boily. 2010. HIV transmission risk through anal intercourse: systematic review, meta-analysis and implications for HIV prevention. *International Journal of Epidemiology* 39 (4): 1048–1063.

Bailey, R.C., S. Moses, C.B. Parker, K. Agot, L. Maclean, J.N. Krieger, C.F.M. Williams, R.T. Campbell, and J.O. Ndinya-Achola. 2007. Male circumcision for HIV prevention in young men in Kisumu, Kenya: a randomised controlled trial. *The Lancet* 369: 643–656.

Balato, N., M. Scalvenzi, S. La Bella, and L. Di Costanzo. 2009. Zoon's balanitis: benign or premalignant lesion? *Case Reports in Dermatology* 1 (1): 7–10.

Bartholomew, S., M. Boscoe, B. Chalmers, S. Dzakpasu, D. Fell, M. Heaman, M.E. Johnston, et al. 2011. *What mothers say: the Canadian maternity experiences survey.* Public Health Agency of Canada.

Bartman, Thomas. 2001. Letter to the editor: Newborn circumcision and urinary tract infections. *Pediatrics* 107 (1): 210.

Bavinton, B.R., A.N. Pinto, N. Phanuphak, B. Grinsztejn, G.P. Prestage, I.B. Zablotska-Manos, J. Fengyi, et al. 2018. Viral suppression and HIV transmission in serodiscordant male couples: an international, prospective, observational, cohort study. *The Lancet HIV* 5 (8): PE438–E447.

Bensley, G.A. and G.J. Boyle. 2003. Effects of male circumcision on female arousal and orgasm. *The New Zealand Medical Journal* 116 (1181): U595.

Berdeu, D., L. Sauze, P. Ha-Vinh, and C. Blum-Boisgard. 2001. Cost-effectiveness of treatments for phimosis: a comparison of surgical and medicinal approaches and their economic effect. *British Journal of Urology International* 87: 239–244.

Beres, Derek. 2016. "Obama signs first anti-persecution legislation protecting atheists." *Big Think*, December 26, 2016. https://bigthink.com/21st-century-spirituality/obama-signs-first-anti-persecution-legislation-protecting-atheists

Bird, S.J. and P.M Hanno. 1998. Bulbocavernosus reflex studies and autonomic testing in the diagnosis of erectile dysfunction. *Journal of the Neurological Sciences* 154 (1): 8–13.

Biryabarema, Elias. 2012. "Uganda says wants to pass anti-gay law as 'Christmas gift.'" *Reuters*, November 13, 2012. https://www.reuters.com/article/us-uganda-homosexuality/uganda-says-wants-to-pass-anti-gay-law-as-christmas-gift-idUSBRE8AC0V720121113

Bishai, D., Y.T. Bonnenfant, M. Darwish, T. Adam, H. Bathija, E. Johansen, and D. Huntington. 2010. Estimating the obstetric costs of female genital mutilation in six African countries. *Bulletin of the World Health Organization* 88 (4): 281–288.

Bisono, G.M., L. Simmons, R.J. Volk, D. Meyer, T.C. Quinn, and S.L. Rosenthal. 2012. Attitudes and decision making bout neonatal male circumcision in a Hispanic population in New York City. *Clinical Pediatrics* 51 (10): 956–963.

Blank, S., J.E. Myers, P. Pathela, K. Washburn, J.K. Varma, J.L. Hadler, T.A. Farley, and J.A. Schillinger. 2012. Neonatal Herpes Simplex Virus Infection Following Jewish Ritual Circumcisions that Included Direct Orogenital Suction — New York City, 2000–2011. *Centers for Disease Control and Prevention Morbidity and Mortality Weekly Report* 61 (22): 405–409.

Bleustein, C.B., H. Eckholdt, J.C. Arezzo, and A. Melman. 2003. Quantitative somatosensory testing of the penis: optimizing the clinical neurological examination. *The Journal of Urology* 169 (6): 2266–2269.

Bleustein, C.B., J.D. Fogarty, H. Eckholdt, J.C. Arezzo, and A. Melman. 2005. Effect of neonatal circumcision on neurologic sensation. *Urology* 65 (4): 773–777.

Bliss, D.P., P.J. Healey, and J.H.T. Waldhausen. 1997. Necrotizing fasciitis after Plastibell circumcision. *The Journal of Pediatrics* 131 (3): 459–462.

Böhm, M., U. Frieling, and T.A. Luger. 2003. Successful treatment of anogenital lichen sclerosus with topical tacrolimus. *Archives of Dermatology* 139 (7): 922–924.

Bollinger, Dan. 2010. Lost boys: an estimate of U.S. circumcision-related infant deaths. *Journal of Boyhood Studies* 4 (1): 78–90.

Bond, Shea Lita. 1999. State Laws Criminalizing Female Circumcision: A Violation of the Equal Protection Clause of the Fourteenth Amendment? *John Marshall Law Review* 32 (2): 353–380.

Bordwell, David. 2006. *Catechism of the Catholic Church: revised edition*. London: Burns and Oates.

Bossio, J.A., C.F. Pukall, and S.S. Steele. 2016. Examining penile sensitivity in neonatally circumcised and intact men using quantitative sensory testing. *The Journal of Urology* 195 (6): 1848–1853.

Boyle, Gregory J. 2003. Issues associated with the introduction of circumcision into a non-circumcising society. *Sexually Transmitted Infections* 79: 427–428.

——. 2015. Does male circumcision adversely affect sexual sensation, function, or satisfaction? Critical comment of Morris and Krieger (2013). *Advances in Sexual Medicine* 5: 7–12.

Boyle, G.J. and G. Hill. 2011. Sub-Saharan African randomized clinical trials into male circumcision and HIV transmission: Methodological, ethical and legal concerns. *Journal of Law and Medicine* 19 (2): 316–334.

Boyle, G.J., R. Goldman, J.S. Svoboda, and E. Fernandez. 2002. Male circumcision: pain, trauma, and psychosexual sequelae. *Journal of Health Psychology* 7 (3): 329–343.

Brigman, W.E. 1985. Circumcision as child abuse: the legal and constitutional issues. *Journal of Family Law* 23 (3): 337–357.

Bristow, E.J. 1977. *Vice and Vigilance: Purity Movements in Britain since 1700*. Gill & Macmillan.

British Medical Association. 2004. The law and ethics of male circumcision: guidance for doctors. *Journal of Medical Ethics* 30: 259–263.

Brody S. and J.J. Potterat. 2003. Assessing the role of anal intercourse in the epidemiology of AIDS in Africa. *International Journal of STD & AIDS* 14: 431–436.

Bronselaer, G.A., J.M. Schober, H.F. Meyer-Bahlburg, G. T'Sjoen, R. Vlietinck, and P.B. Hoebeke. 2013. Male circumcision decreases penile sensitivity as measured in a large cohort. *British Journal of Urology International* 111 (5): 820–827.

Brotherton, J.M.L., M. Fridman, C.L. May, G. Chappell, A.M. Saville, and D.M. Gertig. 2011. Early effect of the HPV vaccination programme on cervical abnormalities in Victoria, Australia: an ecological study. *The Lancet* 377 (9783): 2085–2092.

Brown, M.S., and C.A. Brown. 1987. Circumcision decision: prominence of social concerns. *Pediatrics* 80 (2): 215–219.

Bundesgesetzblatt 2012, Teil I, Nr. 61, 2749. For an English translation, see Section 1631d: http://www.gesetze-im-internet.de/englisch_bgb/englisch_bgb.html#p5744

Bunker, Christopher Barry. 2011. Comments on the British Association of Dermatologists' guidelines for the management of lichen sclerosus 2010. *British Journal of Dermatology* 164 (4): 894–895.

Bunker, C.B., and T.M. Shim. 2015. Male genital lichen sclerosus. *Indian Journal of Dermatology* 60 (2): 111–117.

Camille, C.J., R.L. Kuo, and J.S. Wiener. 2002. Caring for the uncircumcised penis: What parents (and you) need to know. *Contemporary Pediatrics* 19 (11): 61–73.

Campo-Flores, Arian. 2014. "Circumcision coverage comes into focus." *The Wall Street Journal*, January 20, 2014. https://www.wsj.com/articles/SB1000142405270230441 9104579327013566659736

Canfield, J.A. 2001. Letter to the editor: Newborn circumcision and urinary tract infections. *Pediatrics* 107 (1): 212–213.

Carey, A.J., and S.S. Long. 2010. *Staphylococcus aureus*: a continuously evolving and formidable pathogen in the neonatal intensive care unit. *Clinics in Perinatology* 37 (3): 535–546.

Carlisle, Corey G. 2016. The experience of foreskin restoration: a case study. *Journal of Psychology and Christianity* 35 (1): 83–88.

Carmack, A., L. Notini. and B.D. Earp. 2015. Should surgery for hypospadias be performed before an age of consent? *Journal of Sex Research* 53 (8): 1047–1058.

Castellsagué, X., X. Bosch, N. Muñoz, C. Meijer, V.S. Keerti, S.D. Sanjosé, J. Eluf-Neto, et al. 2002. Male circumcision, penile human papilloma virus infection, and cervical cancer in female partners. *New England Journal of Medicine* 346 (15): 1105–1112.

Cathcart, P., M. Nuttall, J. van der Meulen, M. Emberton, and S.E. Kenny. 2003. Trends in paediatric circumcision and its complications in England between 1997 and 2003. *The British Journal of Surgery* 93 (7): 885–890.

Catterall, R.D., and J.K. Oates. 1962. Treatment of balanitis xerotica obliterans with hydrocortisone injections. *British Journal of Venereal Diseases* 38: 75–77.

Center for Disease Control and Prevention. 2010. NCHS Health-E Stat, Trends in circumcision among newborns. February 3, 2010. https://www.cdc.gov/nchs/data/hestat/circumcisions/circumcisions.htm

——. 2014. Recommendations for providers counseling male patients and parents regarding male circumcision and the prevention of HIV, STIs, and other health outcomes. https://beta.regulations.gov/document/CDC-2014-0012-0003

Chambers, Henry F. 2005. Community-associated MRSA: resistance and virulence converge. *The New England Journal of Medicine* 352 (14): 1485–1487.

Chantry, C.J., R.S. Byrd, A.C. Sage, and E.E. Calvert. 2010. Video versus traditional informed consent for neonatal circumcision. *Acta Paediatrica* 99 (9): 1418–1424.

Chessare, John B. 1992. Circumcision: is the risk of urinary tract infection really the pivotal issue? *Clinical Pediatrics* 31 (2): 100–104.

Chung, E., B. Gilbert, M. Perera, and M.J. Roberts. 2015. Premature ejaculation: a clinical review for the general physician. *Australian Family Physician* 44 (10): 737–743.

Cilento, B.G., N.M. Holmes, and D.A. Canning. 1999. Plastibell complications revisited. *Clinical Pediatrics* 38 (4): 239–242.

Cohen, Kerith. 1994. Truth & beauty, deception & disfigurement: a feminist analysis of breast implant litigation. *William and Mary Journal of Women and the Law* 1 (1–7): 149–182.

Cold, Christopher J. 2001. Letter to the editor: Newborn circumcision and urinary tract infections. *Pediatrics* 107 (1): 211.

Cold, C.J., and J.R. Taylor. 1999. The prepuce. *British Journal of Urology* 83 (1): 34–44.

Collins, Dawn. 2014. "Circumcision error leads to Peyronie's disease." *Urology Times,* March 18, 2014. https://www.urologytimes.com/view/circumcision-error-leads-peyronies-disease

Collins, S., J. Upshaw, S. Rutchik, C. Ohannessian, J. Ortenberg, and P. Albertsen. 2002. Effects of circumcision on male sexual function: debunking a myth? *The Journal of Urology* 167 (5): 2111–2112.

Consolini, Deborah M. 2013. Evaluation and care of the normal neonate. *MSD Manual Professional Version.*

Cook, L.S., L.A. Koutsky, and K.K. Holmes. 1994. Circumcision and sexually transmitted diseases. *The American Journal of Public Health* 84 (2): 197–201.

Corbett, H.J., and G.M.E. Humphrey. 2003. Early complications of circumcisions performed in the community. *British Journal of General Practice* 53 (496): 887–888.

Couper, R.T.L. 2000. Methaemoglobinaemia secondary to topical lignocaine/prilocaine in a circumcised neonate. *Journal of Paediatrics and Child Health* 36 (4): 406–407.

CTForum. 2009. "Christopher Hitchens goes after Rabbi Harold Kushner re: Circumcision." YouTube, February 5, 2009. https://www.youtube.com/watch?v=Xx_ov2NiNo4

Darby, Robert. 2003. The masturbation taboo and the rise of routine male circumcision: a review of the historiography. *Journal of Social History* 36 (3): 737–757.

——. 2005. *A Surgical Temptation: The demonization of the foreskin & the rise of circumcision in Britain*. The Chicago University Press.

——. 2011. Infant circumcision in Australia: a preliminary estimate, 2000-10. *Australian and New Zealand Journal of Public Health* 35 (4): 391–392.

——. 2014. Syphilis 1855 and HIV-AIDS 2007: Historical reflections on the tendency to blame human anatomy for the action of micro-organisms. *Global Public Health* 10 (5-6): 573–588.

Darby, Robert, and J. Cozijn. 2013. The British Royal Family's circumcision tradition: genesis and evolution of a contemporary legend. *SAGE Open* 3 (4): 1–10.

Dasgupta, Debarshi. 2011. "The Yin, wounded: a primitive rite for Bohra women sees its first murmurs of protest." *Outlook India*, December 5, 2011. https://www.outlookindia.com/article/the-yin-wounded/279088

Dave, S.S., A. Johnson, K. Fenton, C.H. Mercer, B. Erens, and K. Wellings. 2003. Male circumcision in Britain: findings from a national probability sample survey. *Sexually Transmitted Infections* 79: 499–500.

Davies, Madlen. 2015. "World's first successful penis transplant: Man, 21, has organ restored after it was amputated due to a botched circumcision." *Daily Mail*, March 14, 2015. https://www.dailymail.co.uk/health/article-2993555/World-s-PENIS-transplant-Man-21-organ-restored-amputated-botched-circumcision.html

Davies, Norman. 1996. *Europe: A History*. Oxford University Press, Oxford.

Davis, Dena S. 2001. Male and female genital alteration: a collision course with the law. *Health Matrix* 11: 487–570.

——. 2013. Ancient rites and new laws: how should we regulate religious circumcision of minors? *Journal of Medical Ethics* 0: 1–3.

Dean, R.C., and T.F. Lue. 2005. Physiology of penile erection and pathophysiology of erectile dysfunction. *Urologic Clinics of North America* 32 (4): 379–395.

Dehghankhalili, M., S. Fallahi, F. Mahmudi, F. Ghaffarpasand, M.E. Shahrzad, M. Taghavi, and M. Fereydooni Asl. 2015. Epidemiology, regional characteristics, knowledge, and attitude toward female genital mutilation/cutting in southern Iran. *Journal of Sexual Medicine* 12 (7): 1577–1583.

DeLaet, Debra L. 2009. Framing male circumcision as a human rights issue? Contributions to the debate over the universality of human rights. *Journal of Human Rights* 8 (4): 405–426.

Demirdover, C., B. Sahin, H. Vayvada, and H.Y. Oztan. 2013. Keloid formation after circumcision and its treatment. *Journal of Pediatric Urology* 9: e54–57.

Dickson, N.P., T. Van Roode, P. Herbison, and C. Paul. 2008. Circumcision and risk of sexually transmitted infections in a birth cohort. *Journal of Pediatrics* 152 (3): 383–387.

Dirie, Mahdi A., and Gunilla Lindmark. 1991. Female circumcision in Somalia and women's motives. *Acta Obstetricia et Gynecologica Scandinavica* 70: 581–585.

Dockray, J., A. Finlayson, and G.H. Muir. 2011. Penile frenuloplasty: a simple and effective treatment for frenular pain or scarring. *BJU International* 109 (10): 1546–1550.

Doctors Opposing Circumcision. 2016. "Wrongful foreskin retraction." April 2016. https://www.doctorsopposingcircumcision.org/for-parents/help-with-forcible-foreskin-retraction/

Doerner, R., E. McKeown, S. Nelson, J. Anderson, N. Low, and J. Elford. 2013. Circumcision and HIV infection among men who have sex with men in Britain: the insertive sexual role. *Archives of Sexual Behaviour* 42 (7): 1319–1326.

Douglas, Mary. 1996. *Purity and Danger: An Analysis of Concepts of Pollution and Taboo.* Routledge and Kegan Paul, London.

Dover, Kenneth J. 1989. *Greek Homosexuality.* Cambridge, Massachusetts: Harvard University Press.

Drain, P.K., D.T. Halperin, J.P. Hughes, J.D. Klausner, and R.C. Bailey. 2006. Male circumcision, religion, and infectious disease: an ecologic analysis of 118 developing countries. *BMC Infectious Diseases* 6 (1): 172.

Dube, Gibbs. 2014. "Circumcised men abandoning condoms." *VOA Zimbabwe*, March 5, 2014. https://www.voazimbabwe.com/a/zimbabwe-swaziland-south-africa-medical-male-circumcision-programs/1864352.html

Dunsmuir, W.D., and E.M. Gordon. 1999. The history of circumcision. *British Journal of Urology International* 83 (1): 1–12.

Dwyer, M., N. Peffer, T. Fuller, and G. Cannon. 2016. Intraperitoneal bladder perforation and life-threatening renal failure in a neonate following circumcision with the Plastibell device. *Urology* 89: 134–136.

Earp, Brian D. 2014. Female genital mutilation (FGM) and male circumcision: Should there be a separate ethical discourse? *Practical Ethics.*

——. 2015a. Female genital mutilation and male circumcision: toward an autonomy-based ethical framework. *Medicolegal and Bioethics* 5: 89–104.

——. 2015b. Do the benefits of male circumcision outweigh the risks? A critique of the proposed CDC guidelines. *Frontiers in Pediatrics* 3 (18): 1–6.

——. 2016a. Infant circumcision and adult penile sensitivity: implications for sexual experience. *Trends in Urology and Men's Health* 7 (4): 17–21.

——. 2016b. Science cannot determine human values. *Think* 15 (43): 17–23.

Eason, J.D., M. McDonnell, and G. Clark. 1994. Male ritual circumcision resulting in acute renal failure. *British Medical Journal* 309 (6955): 660–661.

El-Damanhoury, I. 2013. The Jewish and Christian view of female genital mutilation. *African Journal of Urology* 19: 127–129.

Elseesy, Waseem R. 2014. Female circumcision in non-Muslim females in Africa. *African Journal of Urology* 20 (2): 102–103.

Ember Therapeutics. 2016. "Ember Therapeutics Enhances Regenerative Medicine Pipeline With Acquisition of ICX-RHY/Vavelta™ from Intercytex." *GlobeNewswire*, March 16, 2016. https://globenewswire.com/news-release/2016/03/16/820361/0/en/Ember-Therapeutics-Enhances-Regenerative-Medicine-Pipeline-With-Acquisition-of-ICX-RHY-Vavelta-from-Intercytex.html

Eroğlu, E., O.W. Bastian, H.C. Ozkan, O.E. Yorukalp, and A.K. Goksel. 2009. Buried penis after newborn circumcision. *The Journal of Urology* 181 (4): 1841–1843.

Eternal World Television Network. n.d. "Ecumenical Council of Florence 1438-1445."

Accessed October 23, 2020. https://www.ewtn.com/catholicism/library/ecumenical-council-of-florence-1438-1445-1461

Euringer, Amanda. 2006. "BC Health pays to restore man's foreskin." *The Tyee*, July 25, 2006. https://thetyee.ca/News/2006/07/25/Circumcision

Feder, Barnaby J. 1995. "Dow Corning's bankruptcy: the impact on implant suits." *New York Times*, May 21, 1995. https://www.nytimes.com/1995/05/21/business/spending-it-dow-corning-s-bankruptcy-the-impact-on-omplant-suits.html

Fink, Aaron J. 1986. A possible explanation for heterosexual male infection with AIDS. *New England Journal of Medicine* 315 (18): 1167.

Fink, K.S., C.C. Carson, and R.F. DeVellis. 2002. Adult circumcision outcomes study: effect on erectile function, penile sensitivity, sexual activity and satisfaction. *The Journal of Urology* 167 (5): 2113–2116.

Finklestein, I., and N.A. Silberman. 2001. *The Bible Unearthed: Archaeology's New Vision of Ancient Israel and the Origin of Its Sacred Texts*. Free Press.

Fish, Max, A. Shahvisi, T. Gwaambuka, G.B. Tangwa, D. Ncayiyana, and B.D. Earp. 2020. A new Tuskgee? Unethical human experimentation and Western neocolonialism in the mass circumcision of African men. *Developing World Bioethics* 00: 1–16.

Fistarol, S.K., and P.H. Itin. 2013. Diagnosis and treatment of lichen sclerosus. *American Journal of Clinical Dermatology* 14 (1): 27–47.

Food and Drug Administration 2009. Highlights of prescribing information: EVICEL fibrin sealant (human), initial U.S. approval 2003. https://www.fda.gov/media/81499/download

Foreskin Restoration Intactivist Network. n.d. "Forum: In this together: Grief." https://foreskinrestoration.vbulletin.net/forum/in-this-together/grief

Fox, M., and M. Thomson 2012. The New Politics of Male Circumcision: HIV/AIDS, Health law and Social Justice. *Legal Studies* 32 (2): 255–281.

Freeman, Marc. 2014. "Court hears parents battle over circumcision." Sun Sentinel, July 19, 2014. https://www.sun-sentinel.com/news/fl-xpm-2014-07-19-fl-parents-battle-over-circumcision-20140719-story.html

——. 2015. "Mom signs consent for son's circumcision to get out of jail – but now faces new criminal charge." *Sun Sentinel*, May 22, 2015. https://www.sun-sentinel.com/local/palm-beach/fl-circumcision-mother-court-hearing-20150522-story.html

Freeman, Michael. 2002. *Human Rights*. Polity Press.

Frisch, Morten. 2012. Author's response to: Does sexual function survey in Denmark offer any support for male circumcision having an adverse effect? *International Journal of Epidemiology* 41: 312–314.

Frisch, M., M. Lindholm, and M. Grønbæk, 2011. Male circumcision and sexual function in men and women: a survey-based, cross-sectional study in Denmark. *International Journal of Epidemiology*, 40 (5): 1367–1381.

Frisch, M., and J. Simonsen 2021. Non-therapeutic male circumcision in infancy or childhood and risk of human immunodeficiency virus and other sexually transmitted infections: national cohort study in Denmark. *European Journal of Epidemiology* DOI: 10.1007/s10654-021-00809-6.

Frisch, M., Y. Aigrain, V. Barauskas, R. Bjarnason, S. Boddy, P. Czauderna, R.P.E de Gier, et al. 2013. Cultural bias in the AAP's 2012 technical report and policy statement on male circumcision. *Pediatrics* 131 (4): 796–800.

Gairdner, Douglas. 1949. The fate of the foreskin. *The British Medical Journal* 2 (4642): 1433–1437.

Gallo, Luigi. 2013. Patients affected by premature ejaculation due to glans hypersensitivity refuse circumcision as a potential definitive treatment for their problem. *Andrologia* 46 (4): 349–355.

García-Mesa, Y., J. García-Piqueras, R. Cobo, J. Martín-Cruces, I. Suazo, O. García-Suárez, J. Feito, and J.A. Vega. 2021. Sensory innervation of the human male prepuce: Meissner's corpuscles predominate. *Journal of Anatomy* 239 (4): 892–902.

Gao, J., C. Xu, J. Zhang, C. Liang, P. Su, Z. Peng, K. Shi, et al. 2015. Effects of adult male circumcision on premature ejaculation: results from a prospective study in China. *BioMed Research International* Article ID 417846: 1–7.

Geisheker, John. 2011. "What is the greatest danger for an uncircumcised boy? A doctor's visit can harm your boy." *Psychology Today*, October 23, 2011. https://www.psychologytoday.com/blog/moral-landscapes/201110/what-is-the-greatest-danger-uncircumcised-boy

Gemmel, T., and G.J. Boyle. 2000. "Neonatal circumcision: its long term harmful Effects." In *Understanding Circumcision: A Multidisciplinary Approach to a Multi-Dimensional Problem*, edited by George C. Denniston, Frederick M. Hodges, and Marilyn F. Milos, 241–252. Springer.

George, G., K. Govender, S. Beckett, C. Montague, and J. Frohlich. 2016. Early resumption of sex following voluntary medical male circumcision among school-going males. *PLoS One* 11 (12): e0168091.

Gibeau, A.M. 1998. Female genital mutilation: when a cultural practice generates clinical and ethical dilemmas. *Journal of Obstetric, Gynecologic & Neonatal Nursing* 27 (1): 85–91.

Glick, Leonard B. 2005. *Marked in your flesh: Circumcision from ancient Judea to modern America*. Oxford University Press.

Glover, E. 1929. The 'screening' function of traumatic memories. *The International Journal of Psychoanalysis* 10: 90–93.

Goldman, Ronald. 1997. *Circumcision: The Hidden Trauma*. Vanguard Publications.

——. 1999. The psychological impact of circumcision. *British Journal of Urology International* 83 (1): 93–102.

Goldstein, A.T., and L.J. Burrows. 2007. Surgical treatment of clitoral phimosis caused by lichen sclerosus. *American Journal of Obstetrics and Gynecology* 196 (2): 126.e1–126.e4.

Gollaher, D.L. 1994. From ritual to science: the medical transformation of circumcision in America. *Journal of Social History* 28 (1): 5–36.

Gonzalez, R., and B.M. Ludwikowski. 2010. Chapter 9 Male genital anomalies and diseases. In *Handbook of urological diseases in children*. World Scientific Publishing Company. ISBN 9789814287418

Goyal, N.K. 2011. Complete foreskin removal in adult circumcision: Is it a new direction to definitive cure for premature ejaculation? *Indian Journal of Urology* 27 (4): 562–563.

Gray, J., and V.E. Boston. 2003. Glanular reconstruction and preputioplasty repair for distal hypospadias: a unique day-case method to avoid urethral stenting and preserve the prepuce. *British Journal of Urology International* 91 (3): 268–270.

Gray, R.H., K. Godfrey, D. Serwadda, F. Makumbi, S. Watya, F. Nalugoda, N. Kiwanuka, et al. 2007. Male circumcision for HIV prevention in men in Rakai, Uganda: a randomized trial. *The Lancet* 369 (9562): 657–666.

Greer, D.M., P.C. Mohl, and K.A Sheley. 1982. A technique for foreskin reduction and some preliminary results. *The Journal of Sex Research* 18 (4): 324–330.

Greer, Germaine. 2007. *The Whole Woman*. Black Swan.

Griffiths, D., and J.D. Frank. 1992. Inappropriate circumcision referrals by GPs. *Journal of the Royal Society of Medicine* 85: 324–325.

Grisaru, N., S. Lezer, and R.H. Belmaker. 1997. Ritual female genital surgery among Ethiopian Jews. *Archives of Sexual Behavior* 26 (2): 211–215.

Gust, D.A., R.E. Wiegand, K. Kretsinger, S.N. Sansom, P.T. Kilmarx, B.T. Bartholow, and R.T. Chen. 2010. Circumcision status and HIV infection among MSM: reanalysis of a Phase III HIV vaccine clinical trial. *AIDS* 24 (8): 1135–1143.

Halata, Z., and B.L. Munger. 1986. The neuroanatomical basis for the protopathic sensibility of the human glans penis. *Brain Research* 371 (2): 205–230.

Halperin, D.T., and R.C. Bailey. 1999. Male circumcision and HIV infection: 10 years and counting. *The Lancet* 354 (9192): 1813–1815.

Harding, K., M. Sumner, and M. Cardinal. 2013. A prospective, multicentre, randomised controlled study of human fibroblast-derived dermal substitute (Dermagraft) in patients with venous leg ulcers. *International Wound Journal* 10 (2): 132–137.

Harper, D.M., E.L. Franco, C. Wheeler, D.G. Ferris, D. Jenkins, A. Schuind, T. Zahaf, et al. 2004. Efficacy of a bivalent L1 virus-like particle vaccine in prevention of infection with human papillomavirus types 16 and 18 in young women: a randomized controlled trial. *The Lancet* 364: 1757–1765.

Harper, M., and G. Fowlis. 2007. Management of urinary tract infections in men. *Trends in Urology Gynaecology and Sexual Health* 12 (1): 30–35.

Harris, Sam. 2010. *The Moral Landscape*. Great Britain: Bantam Press.

Harryman, Gary L. 2004. "An analysis of the accuracy of the presentation of the human penis in anatomical source materials." In *Flesh and Blood: Perspectives on the Problem of Circumcision in Contemporary Society*, edited by George C. Denniston, Frederick M. Hodges, and Marilyn F. Milos, 17–26. New York: Springer Science+Business Media.

Hartmann, Wolfram. 2013. Expert Statement: Dr med. Wolfram Hartmann, President of "Berufsverband der Kinder- und Jugendärzte" (professional association of paediatricians) English translation.

Haseena, Lockhat. 1999. A preliminary investigation of the psychological effects of female circumcision (female genital mutilation). PhD thesis, Clinical Psychology, Faculty of Medicine, Department University of Manchester, UK.

Helm, K.F. 1991. Lichen sclerosus et atrophicus in children and young adults. *Pediatric Dermatology* 8 (2): 97–101.

Hemmelgarn, Seth. 2016. "Intactivist Jonathon Conte dead at age 34" *The Bay Area Reporter*, May 18, 2016. https://www.ebar.com/news///246292

Hitchens, Christopher. 2005. "Cut it off: another disgusting religious practice." *Slate*, August 29, 2005. https://www.slate.com/articles/news_and_politics/fighting_words/2005/08/cut_it_off.html

Holman, J.R., E.L. Lewis, and R.L. Ringler. 1995. Neonatal circumcision techniques. *American Family Physician* 52 (2): 511–518.

Hoshi, A., Y. Usui, and T. Terachi. 2008. Penile carcinoma originating from lichen planus on glans penis. *Urology* 71 (5): 816–817.

Hovatta, O., M. Mikkola, K. Gertow, A.M. Strömberg, J. Inzunza, J. Hreinsson, B. Rozell, E. Blennow, M. Andäng, and L. Ährlund-Richter. 2003. A culture system using human foreskin fibroblasts as feeder cells allows production of human embryonic stem cells. *Human Reproduction* 18 (7): 1404–1409.

Hume, David. 1739. *A Treatise of Human Nature*. London: John Noon.

Huntley, J.S., M.C. Bourne, F.D. Munro, and D. Wilson-Storey. 2003. Troubles with the foreskin: one hundred consecutive referrals to paediatric surgeons. *Journal of the Royal Society of Medicine* 96: 449–451.

IBISWorld. 2019. "Plastic surgeons: market research report." March 2019. https://www.ibisworld.com/industry/plastic-surgeons.html

Isaacs, D., S. Fraser, G. Hogg, and H.Y. Li. 2003. *Staphylococcus aureus* infections in Australasian neonatal nurseries. *Archives of Disease in Childhood Fetal and Neonatal Edition* 89: F331–F335.

Iwasaki, Akiko. 2010. Antiviral immune responses in the genital tract: clues for vaccines. *Nature Reviews Immunology* 10 (10): 699–711.

Jackson, Beverley. 1997. *Splendid Slippers: A thousand years of an erotic tradition.* California: Ten Speed Press.

Jacobson, N. 2000. *Cleavage: technology, controversy and the ironies of the man-made breast.* New Jersey: Rutgers University Press.

James, Susan Donaldson. 2012. "Baby dies of herpes in ritual circumcision by orthodox Jews." *ABC News*, March 12, 2012. https://abcnews.go.com/Health/baby-dies-herpes-virus-ritual-circumcision-nyc-orthodox/story?id=15888618

Jameson, D.R., C.L. Celum, L. Manhart, and M.R. Golden. 2010. The association between lack of circumcision and HIV, HSV-2, and other sexually transmitted infections among men who have sex with men. *Sexually Transmitted Diseases* 37 (3): 147–152.

Janssen, P.K.C., S.C. Bakker, H. Réthelyi, A.H. Zwinderman, D.J. Touw, B. Olivier and M.D. Waldinger. 2009. Serotonin transporter promoter region (5-HTTLPR) polymorphism is associated with the intravaginal ejaculation latency time in Dutch men with lifelong premature ejaculation. *The Journal of Sexual Medicine* 6 (1): 276–284.

Jee, L.D., and A.J.W. Millar. 1990. Ruptured bladder following circumcision using the Plastibell device. *British Journal of Urology International* 65 (2): 216–217.

Jern, P., P. Santtila, K. Witting, K. Alanko, N. Harlaar, A. Johansson, B. von der Pahlen, et al. 2007. Premature and delayed ejaculation: genetic and environmental effects in a population-based sample of Finnish twins. *The Journal of Sexual Medicine* 4 (6): 1739–1749.

Jewish Business News. 2016. "Intactivist Jews increasingly vocal in Israel." February 7, 2016. http://jewishbusinessnews.com/2016/02/07/intactivist-jews-increasingly-vocal-in-israel

Kaplan, George W. 1983. Complications of circumcision. *Urologic Clinics of North America* 10 (3): 543–549.

Kaplan, Sarah. 2015. "'Intactivism': Why a Florida mother took her son into hiding to avoid circumcision." *The Washington Post*, May 26, 2015. https://www.washingtonpost.com/news/morning-mix/wp/2015/05/26/intactivism-why-a-fla-mother-took-her-son-into-hiding-to-avoid-circumcision/?postshare=5211487077684124&tid=ss_fb&utm_term=.9636eb52cf15

Karim, S.S.A., and R. Gita 1998. Anal sex and HIV transmission in women. *American Journal of Public Health* 88 (8): 1265–1266.

Kayaba, H., H. Tamura, S. Kitajima, Y. Fujiwara, and T. Kato. 1996. Analysis of the shape and retractability of the prepuce in 603 Japanese boys. *Journal of Urology* 156: 1813–1815.

Kearney, S., A. Sharathkumar, and V. Rodriguez. 2015. Neonatal circumcision in severe haemophilia: a survey of paediatric haematologists at United States Hemophilia Treatment Centers. *Haemophilia* 21 (1): 52–57.

Kellogg, John Harvey. 1888. *Treatment for Self-Abuse and its Effects. Plain Facts for Young and Old*. Burlington, Iowa: F Segner & Co.

Kelly, E.J., G. Terenghi, A. Hazari, and M. Wiberg. 2005. Nerve fibre and sensory end organ density in the epidermis and papillary dermis of the human hand. *British Journal of Plastic Surgery* 58: 774–779.

Kigozi. G., M. Wawer, A. Ssettuba, J. Kagaayi, F. Nalugoda, S. Watya, F. Mangen, et al. 2009. Foreskin surface area and HIV acquisition in Rakai, Uganda (size matters). *AIDS* 23 (16): 2209–2213.

Kigozi, G., S. Watya, C.B. Polis, D. Buwembo, V. Kiggundu, M.J. Wawer, D. Serwadda, et al. 2008. The effect of male circumcision on sexual satisfaction and function, results from a randomized trial of male circumcision for human immunodeficiency virus prevention, Rakai, Uganda. *British Journal of Urology International* 101: 65–70.

Kim, D., and M.G. Pang. 2007. The effect of male circumcision on sexuality. *British Journal of Urology International* 99 (3): 619–622.

Kim, D., S. Koo, and M. Pang. 2012. Decline in male circumcision in South Korea. *BMC Public Health* 12: 1067.

Knight, Ernest Jr. 1976. Interferon: purification and characterization from human diploid cells. *Proceedings of the National Academy of Sciences USA* 73 (2): 520–523.

Kojima, N., and J.D. Klausner. 2016. Is emtricitabine-tenofovir disoproxil fumarate pre-exposure prophylaxis for the prevention of human immunodeficiency virus infection safer than aspirin? *Open Forum Infectious Diseases* 3 (1): 1–5.

Kon, M. 1983. A rare complication following circumcision: the concealed penis. *Journal of Urology* 130: 573–574.

Koutsky, L.A., K.A. Ault, C.M. Wheeler, D.R. Brown, E. Barr, F.B. Alvarez, L.M. Chiacchierini, and K.U. Jansen. 2002. A controlled trial of a human papillomavirus type 16 vaccine. *The New England Journal of Medicine* 347: 1645–1651.

Krieger, J.N., S.D. Mehta, R.C. Bailey, K. Agot, J.O. Ndinya-Achola, C.B. Parker, and S. Moses. 2008. Adult Male Circumcision: Effects on Sexual Function and Sexual Satisfaction in Kisumu, Kenya. *Journal of Sexual Medicine* 5 (11): 2610–2622.

Krill, A.J., L.S. Palmer, and J.S. Palmer. 2011. Complications of circumcision. *The Scientific World JOURNAL* 11: 2458–2468.

Kroft, J., and M. Shier. 2012. A novel approach to the surgical management of clitoral phimosis. *Journal of Obstetrics & Gynaecology Canada* 34 (5): 465–471.

Ku, J.H., M.E. Kim, M.K. Lee, and Y.H. Park. 2003. Circumcision practice patterns in South Korea: community based survey. *Sexually Transmitted Infections* 79: 65–67.

Kulkarni, R., and J. Lusher. 2001. Perinatal management of newborns with haemophilia. *British Journal of Haematology* 112 (2): 264–274.

Kwak, C., S. Oh, A. Lee, and H. Choi. 2004. Effect of circumcision on urinary tract infection after successful antireflux surgery. *British Journal of Urology International* 94 (4): 627–629.

Lackey, J.T., R.A. Mannion, and J.E. Kerr. 1968. Urethral fistula following circumcision. *Journal of the American Medical Association* 206 (10): 2318.

Lal, L., J. Audsley, D.A. Murphy, C.K. Fairley, M. Stoove, N. Roth, B.K. Tee, et al. 2017. Medication adherence, condom use and sexually transmitted infections in Australian preexposure prophylaxis users. *AIDS* 31: 1709–1714.

Langton, Helen Elizabeth. 2015. Paediatric anaesthesia: an overview. *Nursing Standard* 30 (9): 52–59.

Larke, N.L., S.L. Thomas, I. dos Santos Silva, and H.A. Weiss. 2011. Male circumcision and penile cancer: a systematic review and meta-analysis. *Cancer*

Causes Control 22: 1097–1110.

Lauder, Jo. 2016. "Labia escape censorship, body image doco MA15+ rating overturned." *Triple J Hack, ABC,* October 18, 2016. https://www.abc.net.au/triplej/programs/hack/is-this-the-end-of-airbrushed-vulvas-in-australian-media/7943676

Leal-Khouri, S., and G.J. Hruza. 1994. Squamous cell carcinoma developing within lichen planus of the penis. Treatment with Mohs' micrographic surgery. *Journal of Dermatologic Surgery and Oncology* 20 (4): 272–276.

Learman, Lee A. 1999. Neonatal circumcision: a dispassionate analysis. *Clinical Obstetrics and Gynecology* 42 (4): 849–859.

Levenson, Jon D. 1993. *The Death and Resurrection of the Beloved Son: The Transformation of Child Sacrifice in Judaism and Christianity.* New Haven: Yale University Press.

Lever, H., D. Ottenheimer, J. Teysir, E. Singer, and H.G. Atkinson. 2018. Depression, anxiety, post-traumatic stress disorder and a history of pervasive gender-based violence among women asylum seekers who have undergone female genital mutilation/cutting: a retrospective case review. *Journal of Immigrant and Minority Health* July 2018 1–7.

Lightfoot-Klein, H. 1991. Prisoners of Ritual: Some Contemporary Developments in the History of Female Genital Mutilation. *Second International Symposium on Circumcision in San Francisco,* Apr 30 – May 3.

Lindboe, A., F. Malmberg, M.K. Aula, F.P. Larsen, M.M. Sigurðardóttir, A.C. Larsen, H. Skari, et al. 2013. Let the boys decide on circumcision: Joint statement from the Nordic Ombudsmen for Children and pediatric experts. Oslo. https://archive.crin.org/en/docs/English-statement-.pdf

Lipscombe, T.K., J. Wayte, F. Wojnarowska, P. Marren and G. Luzzi. 1997. A study of the aetiological factors and possible associations of lichen sclerosus in males. *Australasian Journal of Dermatology* 38 (3): 132–136.

Little, B., and M. White. 2005. Treatment options for paraphimosis. *The International Journal of Clinical Practice* 59 (5): 591–593.

Llewellyn, David J. 1995. Legal remedies for penile torts. *The Compleat Mother* 40: 16.

Lutfi al-Sabbagh, M. 1996. Islamic ruling on male and female circumcision. World Health Organization, Regional Office for the Eastern Mediterranean, Alexandria, Egypt. ISBN 92-9021-216-0.

Lyons, Barry. 2013. Male infant circumcision as a 'HIV vaccine'. *Public Health Ethics* 6 (1): 90–103.

Machan, Tibor R. 2008. Why moral judgements can be objective. *Social Philosophy and Policy* 25 (1): 100–125.

Mack, Edward. 1915. "Chronology of the Old Testament." In *The International Standard Bible Encyclopedia,* edited by James Orr, John Nuelsen, Edgar Mullins, Morris Evans, and Melvin G. Kyle, 18–22. Chicago: The Howard-Severance Company.

Maeda, J.L., R. Chari, and A. Elixhauser. 2012. Circumcisions performed in U.S. community hospitals, 2009. *Agency for Healthcare Research and Quality* Statistical brief #126.

Maimonides, Moses. 1904. *The Guide for the Perplexed.* Translated from the original Arabic text by Michael Friedlaender, 4th revised ed. New York: E.P. Dutton & Company.

Maines, Rachel P. 1999. The technology of orgasm: "hysteria," the vibrator, and women's sexual satisfaction. *The John's Hopkins University Press.*

Mandela, Nelson. 1994. *Long Walk to Freedom: The autobiography of Nelson Mandela.*

London: Abacus.

Marranci, Gabriele. 2014. Female circumcision in multicultural Singapore: the hidden cut. *The Australian Journal of Anthropology* 26 (2): 276–292.

Marshall, Warwick. 2012. *Non-Therapeutic Male Circumcision. Tasmania Law Reform Institute* (Final Report No. 17).

McCormack, S., D.T. Dunn, M. Desai, D.I. Dolling, M. Gafos, R. Gilson, A.K. Sullivan, et al. 2016. Pre-exposure prophylaxis to prevent the acquisition of HIV-1 infection (PROUD): effectiveness results from the pilot phase of a pragmatic open-label randomised trial. *The Lancet* 387: 53–60.

McDonald, Timothy. 2010. "Doctors consider 'less severe' female circumcision." *ABC News*, May 28, 2010. https://www.abc.net.au/news/2010-05-28/doctors-consider-less-severe-female-circumcision/844726

Meeuwis, K.A.P., J.A. De Hullu, L.F.A.G. Massuger, P.C. van de Kerkhof and M.M. van Rossum. 2011. Genital psoriasis: a systematic literature review on this hidden skin disease. *Acta Dermato-Venereologica* 91: 5–11.

Merkel, R., and H. Putzke. 2013. After Cologne: male circumcision and the law Parental right, religious liberty or criminal assault? *Journal of Medical Ethics* 39: 444–449.

Merli, Claudia. 2008. Sunat for girls in Southern Thailand: its relation to traditional midwifery, male circumcision, and other obstetric practices. *Finish Journal of Ethnicity and Migration* 3 (2): 32–41.

Merrill, C.T., M. Nagamine, and C. Steiner. 2008. Circumcisions performed in U.S. community hospitals, 2005. *Agency for Healthcare Research and Quality* Statistical brief #45.

Merritt, Diane F. 2011. Genital trauma in prepubertal girls and adolescents. *Current Opinion in Obstetrics and Gynecology* 23 (5): 307–314.

Midgley, Mary. 1993. "Trying out One's New Sword." In *Vice and Virtue in Everyday Life*, edited by Christina H. Sommers and Fred Sommers, 159–165. Fort Worth: Harcourt Brace Jovanovich College Publishers.

Mihssin, N., K. Moorthy, and P.W.J. Houghton. 1999. Retention of urine: an unusual complication of the Plastibell device. *British Journal of Urology International* 84 (6): 745.

Mill, John Stuart. 1859. *On Liberty*. (4th edition). London: Longman, Roberts & Green Co. Chapter 1.9.

Millett, G. A., H. Ding, J. Lauby, S. Flores, A. Stueve, T. Bingham, A. Carballo-Dieguex, et al. 2007. Circumcision status and HIV infection among Black and Latino men who have sex with men in 3 US cities. *Journal of Acquired Immune Deficiency Syndromes* 46 (5): 643–650.

Mishra, V.C., and H.G. Motiwala. 2010. "Hypospadias." In *Handbook of Pediatric Surgery*, edited by Chandrasen K. Sinha and Mark Davenport, 307–312. Springer.

Misra, S., A. Chaturvedi and N. Misra. 2004. Penile carcinoma: a challenge for the developing world. *The Lancet Oncology* 5 (4): 240–247.

Moldwin, R.M., and E. Valderrama. 1989. Immunochemical analysis of nerve distribution patterns within prepucial tissue. *Journal of Urology* 141 (4): Part 2, p. 499A.

Money, John. 1991. Sexology, body image, foreskin restoration, and bisexual status. *The Journal of Sex Research* 28 (1): 145–156.

Morris, B.J., and T.E. Wiswell. 2013. Circumcision and lifetime risk of urinary tract infection: a systematic review and meta-analysis. *Journal of Urology* 189 (6): 2118–2124.

Morris, B.J., R.G. Wamai, E.B. Henebeng, A.A.R. Tobian, J.D. Klausner, J. Banerjee, and C.A. Hankins. 2016. Estimation of country-specific and global prevalence of male circumcision. *Population Health Metrics* 14 (4): 1–13.

Mulongo, P., C.H. Martin, and S. McAndrew. 2014. The psychological impact of female genital mutilation/cutting (FGM/C) on girls/women's mental health: a narrative literature review. *Journal of Reproductive and Infant Psychology* 32 (5): 469–485.

Munger, B.L., and C. Ide. 1988. The structure and function of cutaneous sensory receptors. *Archives of Histology and Cytology* 51 (1): 1–34.

Munro, N.P., H. Khan, N.A. Shaikh, I. Appleyard, and P. Koenig. 2008. Y-V preputioplasty for adult phimosis: a review of 89 cases. *Urology* 72 (4): 918–920.

Nahm, W.K., L. Zhou, and V. Falanga. 2002. Sustained ability for fibroblast outgrowth from stored neonatal foreskin: a model for studying mechanisms of fibroblast outgrowth. *Journal of Dermatological Science* 28 (2): 152–158.

Nagesh, Ashitha. 2016. "Surgeons sever 10-year-old boy's penis in botched circumcision." *Metro.co.uk*, December 27, 2016. https://metro.co.uk/2016/12/27/surgeons-sever-10-year-old-boys-penis-in-botched-circumcision-6346579/?fb_comment_id=934295180003692_934352396664637#f251986013e8838

National Health Service Inform. 2020. "Penile cancer: About penile cancer." Last revised February 13, 2020. https://www.nhsinform.scot/illnesses-and-conditions/cancer/cancer-types-in-adults/penile-cancer

Naughton, G., J. Mansbridge, and G. Gentzkow. 1997. A metabolically active human dermal replacement for the treatment of diabetic foot ulcers. *International Society for Artificial Organs* 21 (11): 1203–2010.

Nayan, M., R.J. Hamilton, D.N. Juurlink, P.C. Austin, and K.A. Jarvi. 2021. Circumcision and risk of HIV among males from Ontario, Canada. *Journal of Urology* DOI: 10.1097/JU.0000000000002234.

Neill, S.M., F.M. Lewis, F.M. Tatnall, and N.H. Cox. 2010. British Association of Dermatologists' guidelines for the management of lichen sclerosus 2010. *British Journal of Dermatology* 163 (4): 672–682.

Newman, Stephen A. 2016. Why Moses did not circumcise his son. *Jewish Bible Quarterly* 44 (1): 50–52.

News.com.au. 2016. "9-year-old loses penis after circumcision mishap." *New York Post*, December 30, 2016. https://nypost.com/2016/12/30/9-year-old-loses-penis-after-circumcision-mishap

Nguyen, D.M., E. Bancroft, L. Mascola, R. Guevara, and L. Yasuda. 2007. Risk factors for neonatal methicillin-resistance *Staphylococcus aureus* in a well-infant nursery. *Infection Control and Hospital Epidemiology* 28 (4): 406–411.

Nocirc, A. 2011. "Soraya Mire on male and female genital mutilation." *YouTube*, January 16, 2011. https://www.youtube.com/watch?v=Ggqa6CCTR-4

Odemis, E., F.M. Sommez, and Y. Aslan, 2004. Toxic methemoglobinemia due to prilocaine injection after circumcision. *International Pediatrics* 19 (2): 96–97.

Office of the Senior Coordinator for International Women's Issues. 2001. *Indonesia: report on female genital mutilation (FGM) or female genital cutting* (FGC). United States Department of State.

O'Hara, K., and J. O'Hara 1999. The effect of male circumcision on the enjoyment of the female sexual partner. *British Journal of Urology International* 83 (1): 79–84.

Okeke, L.I., A.A. Asinobi, and O.S. Ikuerowo. 2006. Epidemiology of complications of male circumcision in Ibadan, Nigeria. *BMC Urology* 6: 21.

Onyulo, Tonny. 2018. "'This painful practice should be stopped': Teen girls decry painful illegal 'circumcision'." *USA Today*, January 18, 2018. https://www.usatoday.com/story/news/world/2018/01/18/kenya-female-genital-mutilation/1041960001/

Oredsson, Ellen. 2015. "Why do old statues have such small penises?" *How to Talk About Art History*, August 30, 2015. https://www.howtotalkaboutarthistory.com/reader-questions/why-do-all-old-statues-have-such-small-penises

Ornellas, P., and A.A. Ornellas. 2018. HPV vaccination is fundamental for reducing or eradicate penile cancer | Opinion NO. *International Brazilian Journal of Urology* 44 (5): 862–864.

Orsola, A., J. Caffaratti, and J.M. Garat. 2000. Conservative treatment of phimosis in children using a topical steroid. *Urology* 56 (2): 307–310.

Örtqvist, L., M. Fossum, M. Andersson, A. Nordenström, L. Frisén, G. Holmdahl, and A. Nordenskjöld 2016. Sexuality and fertility in men with hypospadias; improved outcome. *Andrology* 5 (2): 286–293.

Osborn, L.M., T.J. Metcalf, and M. Mariani. 1981. Hygienic care in uncircumcised infants. *Pediatrics* 67 (3): 365–367.

Oster, Jakob. 1968. Further fate of the foreskin. *Archives of Disease in Childhood* 43: 400–403.

Paick, J.S., H. Jeong, and M.S. Park. 1998. Penile sensitivity in men with premature ejaculation. *International Journal of Impotence Research* 10 (4): 247–250.

Pang, M.G., and D.S. Kim. 2002. Extraordinarily high rates of male circumcision in South Korea: history and underlying causes. *British Journal of Urology International* 89: 48–54.

Paterson, Tony. 2012. "Germany's Jews and Muslims 'outraged' as circumcision is ruled to cause bodily harm and infringe child's rights." *The Independent*, June 27, 2012. https://www.independent.co.uk/news/world/europe/germany-s-jews-and-muslims-outraged-as-circumcision-is-ruled-to-cause-bodily-harm-and-infringe-7893302.html

Payne, K., L. Thaler, T. Kukkonen, S. Carrier, and Y. Binik. 2007. Sensation and sexual arousal in circumcised and uncircumcised men. *Journal of Sexual Medicine* 4 (3): 667–674.

Pelton, Stephen I. 2009. Circumcision and MRSA. (Expert Opinion). *Factiva*. 40 (10): ISSN: 0037–6337.

Persad, R., S. Sharma, J. McTavish, C. Imber, and P.D. Mouriquand. 1995. Clinical presentation and pathophysiology of meatal stenosis following circumcision. *British Journal of Urology* 75 (1): 91–93.

Piero, L., and A. Alei. 2008. T09-O-39 Surgical treatment of phimosis of the clitoris in woman presenting sexual dysfunction: a case report. *Sexologies* 17 (1): S129.

Podnar, Simon. 2012. Clinical elicitation of the penilo-cavernosus reflex in circumcised men. *British Journal of Urology International* 109 (4): 582–585.

Ponsky, L.E., J.H. Ross, N. Knipper, and R. Kay. 2000. Penile adhesions after neonatal circumcision. *The Journal of Urology* 164 (2): 495–496.

Pope Benedict XVI. 2007. "General audience." *Libreria Editrice Vaticana*, January 31, 2007. https://w2.vatican.va/content/benedict-xvi/en/audiences/2007/documents/hf_ben-xvi_aud_20070131.html

Pope Paul VI. 1965. "Declaration on the relation of the Church to non-Christian religions: Nostra Aetate." *La Santa Sede*, October 28, 1965. https://www.vatican.va/archive/hist_councils/ii_vatican_council/documents/vat-ii_decl_19651028_nostra-aetate_en.html

Porche, Demetrius J. 2006. Paraphimosis: an emergency condition. *The Journal for Nurse Practitioners* 2 (8): 506–507.

Porter, W.M., and C.B. Bunker. 2001. The dysfunctional foreskin. *International Journal of STD & AIDS* 12 (4): 216–220.

Powell, J.J., and F. Wojnarowska. 1999. Lichen sclerosus. *The Lancet* 353 (9166): 1777–1783.

Queensland Law Reform Commission. 1993. Circumcision of Male Infants. Miscellaneous Paper 6: 38–39.

Rajan, P., S.A. McNeill, and K.J. Turner. 2006. Is frenuloplasty worthwhile? A 12-year experience. *Annals of the Royal College of Surgeons of England* 88 (6): 583–584.

Ramjee, G., and E. Gouws. 2002. Prevalence of HIV among truck drivers visiting sex workers ion KwaZulu-Natal, South Africa. *Sexually Transmitted Diseases* 29 (1): 44–49.

Ramos, S., and G.J. Boyle. 2000. Ritual and medical circumcision among Filipino boys: evidence of post-traumatic stress disorder. *Humanities & Social Science Papers* Paper 114.

Rashid, A., S. Patil, and A. Valimalar. 2010. The practice of female genital mutilation among the rural Malays in north Malaysia. *The Internet Journal of Third World Medicine* 9 (1): 1–8.

Rathmann, W.G. 1959. Female circumcision: indications and a new technique. *GP* 20 (3): 115–120.

Reinert, Sue. 2001. "$80,000 settlement to circumcised boy." *The Patriot Ledger*, January 5, 2001.

Rhinehart, John. 1999. Neonatal circumcision reconsidered. *Transactional Analysis Journal* 29 (3): 215–221.

Richters, J., J. Gerofi, and B. Donovan. 1995. Are condoms the right size(s)? A method for self-measurement of the erect penis. *Venereology* 8 (2): 77–81.

Richters, J., A.M.A. Smith, R.O. de Visser, A.E. Grulich, and C.E. Rissel. 2006. Circumcision in Australia: prevalence and effects on sexual health. *International Journal on STD and AIDS* 17: 547–554.

Rickwood, A.M.K., and J. Walker. 1989. Is phimosis overdiagnosed in boys and are too many circumcision performed as a consequence? *Annals of the Royal College of Surgeons of England* 71: 275–276.

Risser, J.M.H., W.L. Risser, M.A. Eissa, P.F. Cromwell, M.S. Barratt, and A. Bortot. 2004. Self-assessment of circumcision status by adolescents. *American Journal of Epidemiology* 159 (11): 1095–1097.

Rizvi, S.A.H., S.A.A. Naqvi, M. Hussain, and A.S. Hasan. 1999. Religious circumcision: a Muslim view. *BJU International* 83 (1): 13–16.

Roberts, Lesley. 2021. *A is for Alex: A Bereaved Mother's Promise to Her Beloved Son.* Great Britain: Cherish Editions.

Robinson, J.L., J.C. Finlay, M.E. Lang, and R. Bortolussi. 2014. Urinary tract infections in infants and children: Diagnosis and management. *Paediatrics and Child Health* 19 (6): 315–325.

Rodger, A.J., V. Cambiano, T. Bruun, P. Vernazza, P. Collins, J. van Lunzen, G.M. Corbelli, et al. 2016. Sexual activity without condoms and risk of HIV transmission in serodifferent couples when the HIV-positive partner is using suppressive antiretroviral therapy. *JAMA* 316 (2): 171–181.

Rodriguez, Sarah W. 2008. Rethinking the history of female circumcision and the clitoridectomy: American medicine and female sexuality in the late nineteenth century. *Journal of the History of Medicine and Allied Sciences* 63 (3): 323–347.

Rodriguez, V., R. Titapiwatanakun, C. Moir, K.A. Schmidt, and R.K. Pruthi. 2010. To circumcise or not to circumcise? Circumcision in patients with bleeding disorders.

Haemophilia 16 (2): 272–276.

Rowland, D.L., S.M. Haensel, J.H.M. Blom, and A.K. Slob. 1993. Penile sensitivity in men with premature ejaculation and erectile dysfunction. *Journal of Sex and Marital Therapy* 19 (3): 189–197.

Royal Australasian College of Physicians. 2010. Circumcision of infant males. Paediatrics & Child Health Division, The Royal Australasian College of Physicians, Sydney, New South Wales, Australia.

Rubin, L., and P. Lanzkowsky. 2000. Cutaneous neonatal herpes simplex infection associated with ritual circumcision. *The Pediatric Infectious Disease Journal* 19 (3): 266–268.

Ryan, C.A., and N.N. Finer. 1994. Changing attitudes and practices regarding analgesia for newborn circumcision. *Pediatrics* 94 (2): 230–233.

Sancaktutar, A.A., N. Pembegül, Y. Bozkurt, B. Kolcu, and A. Tepeler. 2011. Multiple circumferential urethrocutaneous fistulae as a rare complication of circumcision and review of literature. *Urology* 77 (3): 728–729.

Sanchez, J., V.G. Sal y Rosas, J.P. Hughes, J.M. Baeten, J. Fuchs, S.P. Buchbinder, B.A. Koblin, M. Casapia, A. Ortiz, and C. Celum. 2011. Male circumcision and risk of HIV infection among men who have sex with men. *AIDS* 25 (4): 519–523.

Schoen, E.J., M. Oehrli, C.J. Colby, and G. Machin. 2000. The highly protective effect of newborn circumcision against invasive penile cancer. *Pediatrics* 105: E36.

Senkomago, V., D.M. Backes, M.G. Hudgens, C. Poole, K. Agot, S. Moses, P.J.F. Snijders, et al. 2015. Acquisition and persistence of human papillomavirus 16 (HPV-16) and HPV-18 among men with high HPV viral load infections in a circumcision trial in Kisumu, Kenya. *The Journal of Infectious Diseases* 211 (5): 811–820.

Senkul, T., C. Iseri, B. Sen, K. Karademir F. Saraçoğlu and D. Erden 2004. Circumcision in adults: effect on sexual function. *Urology* 63 (1): 155–158.

Serour, F., A. Mandelberg, D. Zabeeda, J. Mori, and S. Ezra. 1998. Efficacy of EMLA cream prior to dorsal penile nerve block for circumcision in children. *Acta Anaesthesiologica Scandinavica* 42 (2): 260–263.

Shenoy, S.P., M. Prashanth Kallaje, S. Pritham, B. Narayana, and R. Amrith Raj. 2015. Frenulum Sparing Circumcision: Step-By-Step Approach of a Novel Technique. *Journal of Clinical and Diagnostic Research* 9(12): PC01–PC03.

Sheu, G., L.M. Revenig, and W. Hsiao. 2014. "Physiology of Ejaculation." In *Men's Sexual Health and Fertility: A Clinician's Guide*, edited by John P. Mulhall and Wayland Hsiao, 13–29. Springer.

Shih, C., C.J. Cold, and C.C. Yang. 2013. Cutaneous corpuscular receptors of the human glans clitoris: descriptive characteristics and comparison with the glans penis. *The Journal of Sexual Medicine* 10 (7): 1783–1789.

Shim, T.N., I. Ali, A. Muneer, and C.B. Bunker. 2016. Benign male genital dermatoses. *British Medical Journal* 354 (i4337): 1–11.

Shingleton, H., and C.W. Heath Jr. (1996, February 16) Letter to Peter Rappo of the American Academy of Pediatrics.

Silvestre, J., C.R. Bess, J.T. Nguyen, A.M. Ibrahim, P.P. Patel, and B.T. Lee. 2014. Evaluation of wait times for patients seeking cosmetic and reconstructive breast surgery. Annals of Plastic Surgery 73 (1): 16–18.

Sivakumar, B., A.A. Brown, and L. Kangesu. 2004. Circumcision in 'buried penis' – a cautionary tale. Annals of the Royal College of Surgeons of England 86 (1): 35–37.

Slater, R., A. Cantarella, L. Franck, J. Meek, and M. Fitzgerald. 2008. How well do clinical pain assessment tools reflect pain in infants? PLOS Medicine 5 (6): 0928–0933.

Slater, R., L. Cornelissen, L. Fabrizi, D. Patten, J. Yoxen, A. Worley, S. Boyd, J. Meek, and M. Fitzgerald. 2010. Oral sucrose as an analgesic drug for procedural pain in newborn infants: a randomised control trial. *The Lancet* 376 (9748): 1225–1232.

Smith, David. 2015. "Barack Obama in Kenya: 'no excuse' for treating women as second-class citizens." *The Guardian*, July 27, 2015. https://www.theguardian.com/us-news/2015/jul/26/barack-obama-condemns-tradition-women-second-class-citizens-nairobi

Sneppen, I., and J. Thorup. 2016. Foreskin morbidity in uncircumcised males. *Pediatrics* 137 (5): 1–7.

Snodgrass, Warren. 2006. Extensive skin bridging with glans epithelium replacement by penile shaft skin following newborn circumcision. *Journal of Pediatric Urology* 2 (6): 555–558.

Sorrells, M.L., J.L. Snyder, M.D. Reiss, C. Eden, M.F. Milos, N. Wilcox, and R.S. Van Howe. 2007. Fine-touch pressure thresholds in the adult penis. *British Journal of Urology International* 99: 846–689.

Spilsbury, K., J.B. Semmens, Z.S. Wisniewski, and C.D. Holman. 2003. Routine circumcision practice in Western Australia. 1981–1999. *ANZ Journal of Surgery* 73: 610–614.

Svoboda, J.S., P.W. Adler, and R.S. Van Howe 2013. Circumcision is unethical and unlawful. *The Journal of Law, Medicine and Ethics* 44 (2): 263–282.

Svoboda, J.S., and R.S. Van Howe. 2013. Out of step: fatal flaws in the latest AAP policy report on neonatal circumcision. *Journal of Medical Ethics* 39 (7): 434–441.

——. 2014. Circumcision: a bioethical challenge. *Journal of Medical Ethics* 40 (7): e-letter.

Swatek-Evenstein, Mark. 2013. Limits of Enlightenment and the Law - On the Legality of Ritual Male Circumcision in Europe today. *Utrecht Journal of International and European Law* 29 (77): 42–50.

Taddio, A., J. Katz, L. Ilersich, and G. Koren. 1997. Effect of neonatal circumcision on pain response during subsequent routine vaccination. *The Lancet* 349 (9052): 599–603.

Tang, W.S., and E.M. Khoo. 2011. Prevalence and correlates of premature ejaculation in a primary care setting: a preliminary cross-sectional study. *The Journal of Sexual Medicine* 8 (7): 2071–2078.

Taves, D.R. 2002. The intromission function of the foreskin. *Medical Hypotheses* 59 (2): 180–182.

The Catholic Leader. 2002. "Jews do not need conversion." November 17, 2002. https://catholicleader.com.au/news/jews-do-not-need-conversion_38374

The Economist. 2016. "An agonising choice." June 18, 2016. http://www.economist.com/news/leaders/21700658-after-30-years-attempts-eradicate-barbaric-practice-it-continues-time-try-new

The Guardian. 2011. "US plastic surgery statistics: chins, buttocks and breasts up, ears down. Data Blog." https://www.theguardian.com/news/datablog/2011/jul/22/plastic-surgery-medicine

The New York Times Editorial Board. 2015. "In New York, a win and a loss on health." *The New York Times*, September 11, 2015. https://www.nytimes.com/2015/09/12/opinion/in-new-york-a-win-and-a-loss-on-health.html?_r=0

The Pew Global Attitudes Project. 2007. World publics welcome global trade – but not immigration: 47-Nation Pew Global Attitudes Survey. Pew Research Center.

Tiemstra, J.D. 1999. Factors affecting the circumcision decision. *The Journal of the American Board of Family Practice* 12 (1): 16–20.

Tobian, A.A.R., D. Serwadda, T.C. Quinn, G. Kigozi, P.E. Gravitt, O. Laeyendecker, B. Charvat, et al. 2009. Male circumcision for the prevention of HSV-2 and HPV infections and syphilis. *The New England Journal of Medicine* 360 (13): 1298–1309.

Tobian, A.A.R., and R.H. Gray. 2011. Male foreskin and oncogenic human papilloma virus infection in men and their female partners. *Future Microbiology* 6 (7): 739–745.

UNAIDS. 2011. Joint strategic action framework to accelerate the scale-up of voluntary medical male circumcision for HIV prevention in Eastern and Southern Africa: 2012–2016.

United Nations (Commission on Human Rights). 2005. *Report of the Special Rapporteur on the question of torture, Manfred Nowak.* UN Doc E/CN.4/2006/6.

United Nations (Committee on the Rights of the Child). 2007. *General Comment No. 8 (2006): The right of the child to protection from corporal punishment and other cruel or degrading forms of punishment (arts. 19; 28, para. 2; and 37, inter alia).* UN Doc CRC/C/GC/8.

——. 2011. General Comment No. 13 (2011): *The right of the child to freedom from all forms of violence.* UN Doc CRC/C/GC/13.

United Nations (General Assembly). 2003. *Resolution adopted by the General Assembly on 22 December 2003: 58/173. The right of everyone to the enjoyment of the highest attainable standard of physical and mental health.* UN Doc A/RES/58/173.

——. 2011. *Right of everyone to the enjoyment of the highest attainable standard of physical and mental health.* UN Doc A/66/254.

United Nations (Human Rights Committee). 2000. *General Comment No. 28: Article 3 (The equality of rights between men and women.* UN Doc CCPR/C/21/Rev.1/Add.10.

——. 2014. *General Comment No. 35: Article 9 (Liberty and Security of Person).* UN Doc CCPR/C/GC/35.

United Nations (Human Rights Council). 2008. *Report of the Special Rapporteur on torture and other cruel, inhuman or degrading treatment or punishment, Manfred Nowak.* UN Doc A/HRC/7/3.

——. 2010. *Report of the Special Rapporteur on torture and other cruel, inhuman or degrading treatment or punishment, Manfred Nowak. Addendum: Study of the phenomena of torture, cruel, inhuman or degrading treatment or punishment in the world, including assessment of conditions of detention.* UN Doc A/HRC/13/39/Add.5.

——. 2013a. *Report of the Special Rapporteur on torture and other cruel, inhuman or degrading treatment or punishment, Juan E. Méndez.* UN Doc A/HRC/22/53.

——. 2013b. *Report of the Special Rapporteur on freedom of religion or belief, Heiner Bielefeldt: Addendum: Mission to the Republic of Sierra Leone.* UN Doc A/HRC/25/58/Add.1.

——. 2016. *Report of the Special Rapporteur on torture and other cruel, inhuman or degrading treatment or punishment.* UN Doc A/HRC/31/57.

Van Duyn, J., and W.S. Warr. 1962. Excessive penile skin loss from circumcision. *Journal of the Medical Association of Georgia* 51: 394–396.

Van Howe, Robert S. 1998. Cost-effective treatment of phimosis. Pediatrics 102: E43.

——. 1999. Does circumcision influence sexually transmitted diseases?: A literature review. *British Journal of Urology International* 83 (1): 52–62.

——. 2005. Effect of confounding in the association between circumcision status and urinary tract infection. *Journal of Infection* 51 (1): 59–68.

——. 2006. Incidence of meatal stenosis following neonatal circumcision in a primary care setting. *Clinical Pediatrics* 45 (1): 49–54.

——. 2007. Human papillomavirus and circumcision: A meta-analysis. *Journal of Infection* 54: 490–496.

——. 2011. How the circumcision solution in Africa will increase HIV infections. *Journal of Public Health in Africa* 2:e4: 11–15.

——. 2015. A CDC-requested, evidence-based critique of the Centers for Disease Control and Prevention 2014 draft on male circumcision: How ideology and selective science lead to superficial, culturally-biased recommendations by the CDC. DOI: 10.13140/2.1.1148.4964.

Van Howe, R.S., and F.M. Hodges. 2006. The carcinogenicity of smegma: debunking a myth. *Journal of the European Academy of Dermatology and Venereology* 20: 1046–1054.

Villa, L.L., R.L. Costa, C.A. Petta, R.P. Andrade, K.A. Ault, A.R. Giuliano, C.M. Wheeler, et al. 2005. Prophylactic quadrivalent human papillomavirus (types 6, 11, 16, and 18) L1 virus-like particle vaccine in young women: a randomised double-blind placebo-controlled multicentre phase II efficacy trial. *The Lancet Oncology* 6: 271–278.

Volksbegehren gegen Kirchen-Privilegien. 2012. "The consequences can be worse for Boy than for Girl." *YouTube*, October 31, 2012. https://www.youtube.com/watch?v=NaEoQVZnN8I

von Frey M. 1894. Beitraege zur Physiologie des Schmerzsinns. Zweite Mitt. Akad Wiss Leipzig Math Naturwiss Kl Ber 46: 283–296.

Voris, B.R.I., C.D.N. Visintin, and L.O. Reis. 2018. HPV vaccination is fundamental to reducing or eradicate penile cancer | Opinion: YES. *International Brazilian Journal of Urology* 44 (5): 859–861.

WADI. 2010. Female genital mutilation in Iraqi-Kurdistan. WADI, Association for Crisis Assistance and Development Co-operation.

Waldinger, Marcel D. 2002. The neurobiological approach to premature ejaculation. *The Journal of Urology* 168 (6): 2359–2367.

Wamai, R.G., B.J. Morris, J.H. Waskett, E.C. Green, J. Banerjee. R.C. Bailey, J.D. Klausner, D.C. Sokal, and C.A. Hankins. 2012. Criticisms of African trials fail to withstand scrutiny: male circumcision does prevent HIV transmission. *Journal of Law and Medicine* 20: 93–123.

Wan, Julian. 2002. Gomco circumcision clamp: an enduring and unexpected success. *Urology* 59 (5): 790–794.

Wawer, M.J., F. Makumbi, G. Kigozi, D. Serwadda, S. Watya, F. Nalugoda, D. Buwembo, et al. 2009. Circumcision in HIV-infected men and its effect on HIV transmission to female partners in Rakai, Uganda: a randomized control trial. *The Lancet* 374: 229–237.

Warren, John. 2010. "Physical effects of circumcision." In *Genital Autonomy: Protecting Personal Choice*, edited by George C. Denniston, Frederick M. Hodges, and Marilyn F. Milos, 75–79. Springer Science+Business Media.

Weaver, B.A., Q. Feng, K.K. Holmes, N. Kiviat, S.K. Lee, C. Meyer, M. Stern, and L.A. Koutsky. 2004. Evaluation of genital sites and sampling techniques for human papilloma virus DNA in men. *The Journal of Infectious Diseases* 189 (4): 677–685.

Weiss, Charles. 1962. A worldwide survey of the current practice of milah (ritual circumcision). *Jewish Social Studies* 24 (1): 30–48.

Weiss, H.A., S.L. Thomas, S.K. Munabi, and J.J. Hayes 2006. Male circumcision and the risk of syphilis, chancroid, and genital herpes: a systematic review and meta-analysis. *Sexually Transmitted Infections* 82 (2): 101–109.

Wellington, M., and M.J. Rieder. 1993. Attitudes and practices regarding analgesia for newborn circumcision. *Pediatrics* 92 (4): 541–543.

Weisman, Rebecca. 1993. Reforms in medical device regulation: an examination of the silicone gel breast implant debacle. *Golden Gate University Law Review* 23: 973–1000.

Werker P.M., A.A. Terng, and M. Kon. 1998. The prepuce free flap: dissection feasibility study and clinical application of a super-thin new flap. *Plastic and Reconstructive Surgery* 102: 1075–1082.

Williams, Bernard. 1976. *Morality: an Introduction to Ethics.* Cambridge: Cambridge University Press.

Williamson, M.L., and S. Paul. 1988. Women's preference for penile circumcision in sexual partners. *Journal of Sex Education Therapy* 14 (2): 8–12.

Windahl, Torgny. 2006. Is carbon dioxide laser treatment of lichen sclerosus effective in the long run? *Scandinavian Journal of Urology and Nephrology* 40 (3): 208–211.

Winkelmann, R.K. 1956. The cutaneous innervation of the human newborn prepuce. *Journal of Investigative Dermatology* 26 (1): 53–67.

Wong, David. 1993. "Relativism." In *A Companion to Ethics*, edited by Peter Singer, 442–450. Oxford: Blackwell.

World Health Organization. 2007. Male circumcision: Global trends and determinants of prevalence, safety and acceptability. *IWHO Library Cataloguing-in-Publication Data*, ISBN 9789241596169.

——. 2008. Eliminating Female Genital Mutilation: An Interagency Statement: OHCHR, UNAIDS, UNDP, UNECA, UNESCO, UNFPA, UNHCR, UNICEF, UNIFEM, WHO (2008).

——. 2016. *WHO guidelines on the management of health complications from female genital mutilation.* ISBN 978 92 4 154964 6

——. 2018. Care of girl & women living with female genital mutilation: a clinical handbook. Licence: CC BY-NC-SA 3.0 IGO.

Xie, L.H., S.K. Li, and Q. Li. 2013. Combined treatment of penile keloid: a troublesome complication after circumcision. *Asian Journal of Andrology* 15: 575–576.

Xin, Z.C., W.S. Chung, Y.D. Choi, D.H. Seong, Y.J. Choi, and H.K. Choi. 1996. Penile sensitivity in patients with primary premature ejaculation. *The Journal of Urology* 156 (3): 979–981.

Yang, S.S.D., Y.C. Tsai, C.C. Wu, S.P. Liu, and C.C. Wang. 2005. Highly potent and moderately potent topical steroids are effective in treating phimosis: a prospective randomized study. *The Journal of Urology* 173: 1361–1363.

Yildirim, S., T. Akoz, and M. Akan. 2000. A rare complication of circumcision: concealed penis. *Plastic and Reconstructive Surgery* 106 (7): 1662–1663.

Ying, H., and Z. Xiu-hua. 1991. Balloon dilation treatment for phimosis in boys: report of 512 cases. *Chinese Medical Journal* 104 (6): 491–493.

Zampieri, N., M. Corroppolo, F.S. Camoglio, L. Giacomello, and A. Ottolenghi. 2005. Phimosis: stretching methods with or without application of topical steroids? *The Journal of Pediatrics* 147 (5): 705–706.

Zhou, C., X. Jiang, Z. Xu, L. Guo, J. Chen, H. Wang, D. Zhang, and B. Shi. 2010. Bulbocavernosus reflex to stimulation of prostatic urethra in patients with lifeline premature ejaculation. *Journal of Sexual Medicine* 7 (11): 3750–3757.

Zwi Werblowsky, R.J., and G. Wigoder. 1997. Circumcision. In *The Oxford Dictionary of the Jewish Religion.* New York & Oxford: Oxford University Press.

Acknowledgments

I am indebted to Fiona Cooke, Batool Moussa, Idan Ben-Barak, and Travis Wisdom, who all provided feedback on the draft manuscript in its entirety. The manuscript benefited greatly from Fiona's and Batool's editorial eyes, as well as Idan's philosophical and Travis' legal minds.

Travis Wisdom played a critical role in the development of my thinking about human rights and genital autonomy, through our many discussions on the subject, and through the following coauthored work: Meddings, Jonathan, and T.L.C. Wisdom. 2017. *Genital Autonomy*. The Rationalist Society of Australia.

I would also like to thank Marilyn Milos, Georganne Chapin, Brian Earp, Morten Frisch, Robert Darby, and Rabbi Dovid Gutnick for taking the time to answer my questions, Jenny Browne for the book's index, and Anne Donald for the book's cover design, page design, and illustrations of circumcision procedures.

About the author

Jonathan Meddings is an Australian writer and human rights advocate. The author of more than 100 medical fact sheets and coauthor of peer-reviewed scientific papers and market-leading biology textbooks, Jonathan leads The Darbon Institute, a charity working to protect and promote everyone's right to bodily integrity and autonomy in Australia and New Zealand.

Throughout his career as a public policy professional, Jonathan has championed evidence-based health policy and defended the rights of vulnerable people and communities.

Jonathan holds a Bachelor of Medical Laboratory Science with Honours and a Bachelor of Arts with majors in philosophy and politics.

Always quick to get to the point, Jonathan coaches the sport of fencing at Australia's premier fencing club.

Recommended websites

circumcisionbook.com
jonathanmeddings.com

A

abuse, circumcision as 79–80, 83, 118
acquired immunodeficiency syndrome see
   HIV
activism see bodily autonomy movement
adhesions, penile 53
adult circumcision see age...
aesthetics
   aesthetic argument for circumcision
      11–12, 66–67
   anti-intact stigma 67–68, 71
   harm caused by sexual objectification
      66–67
   marketing cosmetic surgery 61–62
   personal subjectivity 64–65
   societal subjectivity 59–61, 66–67
Africa
   female genital mutilation in 102–103
   HIV campaign 8, 25, 27, 38–45
age and foreskin development 17–18, 29
age of circumcision see also bodily
   autonomy movement; legislation
   conformity and 68
   disease and 26, 33, 35–36, 55
   health professionals on 25–27
   human rights and 9–10, 70, 78–85,
      106–110
   hygiene and 34
   hypospadias surgery 36–37
   pain dependent on 26–27, 63
   religion and 9, 77–78, 80–81, 89
   in UNAIDS initiative 42
AIDS see HIV
America
   anti-circumcision movement 105–106,
      115–117
   circumcision deaths 55
   genital cutting legislation 8, 70, 82–83
   history of genital cutting 28
   obtaining consent for circumcision
      105–106
   prevalence of surgery 61–62, 68, 73
American Academy of Pediatrics (AAP)
   15, 25–26, 33, 85
American Cancer Society 33
American Society of Plastic Surgeons
   61–62
amputation 54
anal sex 38–40, 42
Ancient Greece 59

Ancient Rome 59
anesthesia 27–28, 46, 50, 55, 63
antisemitism 77–78, 99–100
appearance see aesthetics
Arab states 90, 103
Association of Pediatricians 78
Aulus Cornelius Celsus 59
Australia 72, 81, 85, 87
autonomy see bodily autonomy movement

B

babies see abuse; age...
bathing 17, 34–35
Benedict XVI, Pope 100
Beyond the Bris 98
Bible 91–92 see also Genesis 17; Leviticus
   12
Bigelow, Jim 57
biotechnology 63–64
bisexuality 38–40, 42
bladder 54
blood loss 51
Bloomberg, Mike 94
bodily autonomy movement 97, 115–118
   see also informed consent; Intact America
body image 56 see also aesthetics
breast augmentation 61–62
bris and brit milah see Judaism and Jewish
   culture
brit shalom 98
Britain 28, 74, 82, 106
British Medical Association 106
Bruchim 98
bulbocavernosus reflex 22–24
bullying 67–68, 71
buried penis 53

C

Canada 55, 72
cancer 31–34
Catholicism 100
Celsus, Aulus Cornelius 59
Centers for Disease Control and
   Prevention (CDC) 26–27, 73
cervical cancer 31–32
Chapin, Georganne 105
Charles, King 74
children see abuse; age...
China 66
Christianity see also Exodus; Genesis 17;

Leviticus 12
  African circumcision practice and 88,
    103
  current views on circumcision 100–
    101
  history of circumcision 98–101
circumcision *see also* aesthetics;
  conformity; genital autonomy
  movement; health; history of genital
  cutting; morality
    complications 50–56
    cost 62–63
    foreskin restoration 56–57
    procedure 12, 46–50, 54
    rates of circumcision 72–75, 101
    use of term 8–9, 12–13
Circumcision Center 62
class 74–75
clitoris and clitoral hood 14, 18, 28, 30–
  31, 60 *see also* female genital mutilation
clotting factors 51
Cologne, Germany 77–78
Committee on the Rights of the Child
  79–80
concealed penis 53
condoms 21–22, 43–44
conformity 11, 66–71 *see also* aesthetics;
  purity and class ideals; rates of
  circumcision; stigma
consent *see* informed consent
Conte, Jonathon 117
contraception 21–22, 43–44
Convention on the Rights of the Child
  79–80
Coptic Christianity 101
corpuscular receptors *see* sensitivity
cost of circumcision 62–63
Council of Europe 82
Council of Jerusalem 98–99
court judgements
  on informed consent 6–7, 77–78,
    82–83, 105
  on surgical errors 54
criminalization of genital cutting 87–88
culture 107–112 *see also* conformity;
  morality; religion

D
The Darbon Institute 87
Darby, Robert 45

de Blasio, Bill 94
De medicina 59
death 52, 55, 94, 117
developing countries 34–35 *see also* HIV
disfigurement 16, 30–31, 52, 54–55
Doctors Opposing Circumcision 18
Douglas, Mary 75
Dover, Kenneth 59

E
Earp, Brian 14, 20
Ecumenical Council of Florence 99
Egypt 101
ejaculation 22–24 *see also* sensitivity
erectile function 16, 22–24
ethics *see* morality
Europe 82
evangelical Christianity 100–101
excision 14, 29
Exodus 91–92

F
fact-value distinction 112–114
*Female Circumcision: Indications and a New
  Technique* 28–29
female foreskin *see* clitoris and clitoral
  hood
female genital mutilation
  adult genital surgery 60–61
  in Africa 101
  compared to male 6–9, 12–15, 82–83,
    118
  history of 28–29, 90
  in Islam 102–103
  legislation on 7–8, 87–88
  proposed legalization of 15, 85–86
  regulation of 79, 81–83
  relativist argument 109–110
  sexual objectives of 60–61, 66
  types of 14–15
females *see* women
fetus development 17
fibrin glue 51
fibroblasts 63–64
Fink, Aaron J. 38
fistula 53–54
foetus development 17
footbinding 66
foreskin *see also* circumcision; clitoris and
  clitoral hood

development 17–18, 29–30
fibroblasts 63–64
functions 16–17
restoration 56–57
frenulum pain and scarring 37
Frisch, Morten 20

G
gangrene 54–55
gay and bisexual men 38–40, 42
gender *see* intersex people; men; women
general anesthesia 27, 63
Genesis 17 90–92, 96, 100
genetics 23
genital autonomy movement 97, 115–118
  see also informed consent; Intact America
genital cutting *see also* circumcision;
  female genital mutilation; hypospadias
  terminology 8–9, 12–13
Gentle Circumcision 63
Germany 77–78, 82
Gillen, Jeffrey Dana 6
Glick, Leonard 95
global rates of circumcision 72–75, 101
Gollaher, David 75
Gomco technique 46–47, 50, 54
Greece 59
Greek Homosexuality 59
Greer, Germaine 109–110

H
hadith 101
Hardy, Alex 117
harm minimisation 15, 85–86
Harry, Prince 74
health 11 *see also* history of genital
  cutting; immunity and inflammation;
  pain; psychological health; sexuality; skin
  damage and skin conditions
    blood loss 51
    buried penis 53
    circumcision deaths 52, 55, 94, 117
    hypospadias 36–37
    importance of wellbeing 113–114
    institutiuonal medical policies 25–27
    kidney failure 54
    meatal stenosis 53–54
    medical necessity 108–109
    methemoglobinemia 55
    phimosis and paraphimosis 29–30, 34

urethral fistula 53–54
Heath, Clark 33
Hebrew Bible 91–92 *see also* Genesis 17;
  Leviticus 12
hemophilia 51
herpes 94
Hironimus family 6–7
Hirsi Ali, Ayaan 15
Hispanic populations 73
history of genital cutting
  in Christianity 98–101
  introduction to medicine 27–29
  in Islam 101–102
  in Judaism 90–97
Hitchens, Christopher 9
HIV
  African campaign against 8, 25, 27,
    38–45
  condom use and medication 43–44
homosexuality 38–40, 42
Howe, Robert Van 20
HSV-1 (herpes simplex virus type 1) 94
human immunodeficiency virus *see* HIV
human papillomavirus (HPV) 31–32
human rights *see* rights
Hume, David 112–113
hygiene 17, 34–35, 75, 103 *see also*
  infections
hypospadias 36–37

I
immunity and inflammation 17, 30–31
  see also infections
incidence of circumcision 72–75, 101
infants *see* abuse; age...
infections 35–36, 51–52, 109 *see also*
  sexually transmitted infections
infibulation 14
inflammation 30–31
informed consent 26, 105–106 *see also*
  age of circumcision; bodily autonomy
  movement
Intact America 105–106
intactness 9 *see also* genital autonomy
  movement; health; stigma
international rates of circumcision 72–75,
  101
International Symposium on Genital
  Autonomy and Children's Rights 116
intersex people 79, 81, 87

Iowa 67

Islam
  circumcision rates within 7, 101
  genital cutting procedure 89, 104
  motivations behind genital cutting in
    101–104
  ritual circumcision court judgements
    77, 82
is-ought problem 112–114

J
Jackson, Beverley 66
Jewish culture *see* Judaism and Jewish
  culture
Joint United Nations Programme on HIV/
  AIDS 25, 27, 39, 42–43
The Joy of Uncircumcising 57
Judaism and Jewish culture *see also*
  Exodus; Genesis 17; Leviticus 12
  antisemitism and circumcision 77–78,
    99–100
  circumcision procedure 89, 92–96,
    104
  legality of ritual circumcision 77–78,
    94
  metzitzah b'peh 93–94
  motivations behind genital cutting in
    95–97
  prevalence of genital cutting 90, 94,
    98, 104

K
Kasper, Walter 100
keloid formation 52
Kenya 8, 20–21, 38–44
kidney failure 54
Kushner, Harold 97

L
labia 60–61 *see* also female genital
  mutilation
legislation *see also* court judgements
  legality of genital cutting 8, 81–83,
    87–88
  logistics of banning 85–88
Leviticus 12 91, 95–96
LGBTQIA 38–40, 42 *see also* intersex
  people
lichen planus and sclerosus 30–31
local anaesthetic 46, 55

Long Walk to Freedom 107–108

M
Maimonides, Moses 96–97
Maines, Rachel 28
males *see* men
Malta 81
Mandela, Nelson 107–108
*Marked in Your Flesh: Circumcision from
  Ancient Judaea to Modern America* 95
marketing 61–62
Mason, Paul 87
masturbation 28, 100
A Measure of his Grief 98
meatal stenosis 53–54
medical effects of circumcision *see* health
medication 43–44, 51–52 *see also*
  anesthesia
men 95–96, 108 *see also* aesthetics;
  foreskin; penis
mental health *see* psychological health
Merkel, Angela 77
methemoglobinemia 55
methicillin 51–52
metzitzah b'peh 93–94
microbes *see* infections
micromastia 62
Middle East 103
Mill, John Stuart 107
Milos, Marilyn 115–116
minors *see* abuse; age...
Mire, Soraya 15
misogyny 95–96, 108
Mogen technique 46, 48, 50
morality 74–75, 103 *see also* informed
  consent; religion; rights
  moral relativism 11, 108–114
mortality rate 52, 55, 94, 117
Moss, Lisa Braver 98
MRSA and MSSA 51–52
Muhammad 101
Muslim culture *see* Islam

N
National Organization of Restoring Men
  (NORM) 57
Nebus-Hironimus family 6–7
necrosis 54–55
neonatal circumcision *see* abuse; age...
New England Journal of Medicine 38

New York City, US 94
Nigeria 50
Nordic Association of Children's
  Ombudsmen 82
Nostra Aetate 100

O
Obama, Barack 8
"Old Dogs, New Dicks" 68
On Liberty 107
Oredsson, Ellen 59
orgasm *see* sensitivity
Orthodox Judaism 94

P
pain *see* also anesthesia
  during circumcision 50, 55–56, 96–97
  post-circumcision 16, 37, 55–56
paraphimosis and phimosis 29–30, 34
parental rights and responsibilities *see*
  rights
Paul (apostle) 99
Paul VI, Pope 100
Pecoraro, Gino 85
Pediatrics 25
penis *see* foreskin; health
PEP and PrEP (post and pre-exposure
  prophylaxis) 43–44
Peter (apostle) 98–99
Pew Research Center 39
philosophy *see* morality
phimosis and paraphimosis 29–30, 34
Plastibell technique 46, 49–50, 54
popularity of circumcision 72–75, 101
pornography 60
post-traumatic stress disorder (PTSD) 56
pre and post-exposure prophylaxis (PrEP
  and PEP) 43–44
pregnancy 17
premature ejaculation 22–24
prevalence of circumcision 72–75, 101
pricking of clitoris 15
protests *see* genital autonomy movement
psychological health 24, 55–56, 116–117
  see also abuse; pain; stigma
purity and class ideals 74–75, 103
*Purity and Danger: An Analysis of Concepts
  of Pollution and Taboo* 75

Q
Queensland Circumcision Service 63
Queensland Law Reform Commission 81
queer identity 38–40, 42 *see also* intersex
  people

R
rates of circumcision 72–75, 101
Rathmann, W. G. 28–29
*Recommendations for providers counseling
  male patients and parents regarding male
  circumcision and the prevention of HIV,
  STIs, and other health outcomes* 26
religion *see also* Christianity; Islam;
  Judaism and Jewish culture
  freedom of religion argument 9, 11,
    76–77, 79–81, 84–85
  legality of religious circumcision 8, 70,
    75, 77–78, 82–83, 88
religious texts 91–92, 101 *see also* Genesis
  17; Leviticus 12
ridged band 56
rights 11, 78–82 *see also* culture;
  informed consent; legislation; religion
ritual circumcision *see* religion
Rome 59
Royal Australasian College of Physicians
  33, 72
The Royal Australian and New
  Zealand College of Obstetricians and
  Gynecologists (RANZCOG) 85
rural areas 73

S
scarring 16, 30–31, 52, 54–55
Schoen, Edgar 74
self-esteem 56 *see also* aesthetics
sensitivity *see also* ejaculation
  incidental reduction via genital cutting
    16, 18–22
  intentional reduction via genital cutting
    22, 28, 97, 100
  mechanisms of 18–19
  studies on 18–22
sex and gender *see* intersex people; men;
  women
Sex and the City 68
sexuality *see also* aesthetics; sensitivity;
  sexually transmitted infections
    condom use 21–22, 43–44

ejaculation 22–24
erectile function and circumcision 16,
     22–24
foreskin's role in penetration 16
homosexuality and bisexuality 38–40,
     42
role in history of circumcision 27–29,
     75, 97, 103
sexual function studies 20–22
sexually transmitted infections 26–27, 45,
     94, 107 *see also* HIV
shaming 67–68, 71
Shingleton, Hugh 33
showering 17, 34–35
skin damage and skin conditions 16–17,
     30–31, 53 *see also* cancer; disfigurement;
     sexually transmitted infections
smegma 34
soap 17, 35
social class 74–75
Somalia 101
South Africa 38–44, 82, 88
South Korea 73–74
*Splendid Slippers: A Thousand Years of An
     Erotic Tradition* 66
squamous cell carcinomas 33
Staphylococcus aureus 51–52
stigma 67–68, 71
STIs (sexually transmitted infections)
     26–27, 45, 94, 107 *see also* HIV
Sudan 101
suicide 117
surgery 36–37, 56–57, 61–62 *see also*
     circumcision; female genital mutilation
syphilis 45

T
Tasmania Law Reform Institute 81
Tinari, Paul 64
tissue death *see* necrosis
topical anaesthetic 46, 55
torture, circumcision as 79–80
touch receptors *see* pain; sensitivity
tradition 103 *see also* conformity
trapped penis 53
Treatise of Human Nature 112–113
tugging method 57

U
Uganda 20–21, 38–44
United Kingdom 28, 74, 82, 106
United Nations
     Convention on the Rights of the Child
          79–80
     UNAIDS 25, 27, 39, 42–45
United States of America *see* America
University of Iowa 71
upper class 74–75
urban areas 73
urethra 36–37, 53–54
urinary tract infections (UTIs) 35–36
urination 36–37, 53–54

V
vaccines 32, 107
vagina 14, 16 *see also* female genital
     mutilation
Van Howe, Robert 20, 39
Vena, Cornel 76
Victoria, Queen 74
Vienna Declaration and Programme of
     Action 78
violence, circumcision as 79–80
voluntary male medical circumcision
     initiative 25, 27, 39, 42–45

W
wellbeing *see* health
WHO (World Health Organization) 7,
     14, 25, 27, 43
The Whole Woman 109–110
William, Prince 74
women 38, 43, 95–97, 108 *see also*
     aesthetics; breast augmentation; cervical
     cancer; clitoris and clitoral hood; female
     genital mutilation; pregnancy; vagina
World Conference on Human Rights 78
     World Health Organization 7, 14, 25,
          27, 43

X
Xhosa tribe 107–108

Z
Zoon's balanitis 31